CLEAN SKIN
FROM WITHIN

The Spa Doctor's **2-Week Program**
to Glowing, Naturally Youthful Skin

Dr. Trevor Cates

FAIR WINDS

Inspiring | Educating | Creating | Entertaining

Brimming with creative inspiration, how-to projects, and useful information to enrich your everyday life, Quarto Knows is a favorite destination for those pursuing their interests and passions. Visit our site and dig deeper with our books into your area of interest: Quarto Creates, Quarto Cooks, Quarto Homes, Quarto Lives, Quarto Drives, Quarto Explores, Quarto Gifts, or Quarto Kids.

Library of Congress Cataloging-in-Publication Data

Cates, Trevor.

Clean skin from within : the spa doctor's two-week program to glowing, naturally youthful skin / Dr. Trevor Cates, the Spa Doctor.

ISBN 9781592337439 (paperback)

1. Skin—Care and hygiene—Popular works.

2. Skin—Diet therapy.

RL87 .C37 2017   646.7/26—dc23

2016035416

Design and page layout: Laura Shaw Design, Inc.

Cover Image: Shutterstock

Photography: Adam Finkle; Shutterstock (pages 8, 16, 18, 31, 50, 52, 54, 72, 87, 97, 111, 129, 172, 175, and 193)

Printed in China

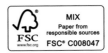

MIX
Paper from responsible sources
FSC® C008047
www.fsc.org

The information in this book is for educational purposes only. It is not intended to replace the advice of a physician or medical practitioner. Please see your health-care provider before beginning any new health program.

21 20 19 18 17   1 2 3 4 5

ISBN: 978-1-59233-922-8

"A guide to better skin and a better you. Dr. Cates teaches readers that diet does matter and that healthy skin comes from within."
—Alan Christianson, N.M.D., *New York Times* best-selling author of *The Adrenal Reset Diet*

"Read this book to learn how the things that will make you live way past 100 can also make you look amazing right now. Dr. Cates will transform how you think about your skin and aging."
—Dave Asprey, best-selling author of *The Bulletproof Diet*

"Dr. Trevor Cates truly understands that healthy and beautiful skin is mostly an INSIDE job! People who have been spending thousands on somewhat dangerous lotions and potions to assist in the aging process can now take control and age gracefully from the inside out."
—Dr. Holly Lucille, N.D., R.N., founder of InherentlyYou.com

"The approach is clear: Get to the root cause for true relief."
—Thaddeus Gala, D.C., Complete Care Health Centers

"Everyone who reads this book will benefit with a relevant takeaway, whether you're trying to heal from a skin condition or simply want to maintain a youthful glow."
—Rachael Pontillo, M.Msc., C.N.A.P., C.I.H.C., L.E., best-selling author of *Love Your Skin, Love Yourself*

"Trevor is a living example of what she shares in her excellent new book, *Clean Skin from Within*. And her healthy recipes are delicious!"
—Mitchell A. Fleisher, M.D., D.Ht., D.A.B.F.M., Dc.A.B.C.T., author of *Alternative DrMCare Natural Medical Self-Care Protocols*

"*Clean Skin from Within* provides a powerful toolbox for anyone ready to reclaim their health and have it radiantly reflected in their well-nourished skin."
—Izabella Wentz, Pharm.D., F.A.S.C.P., pharmacist, and *New York Times* best-selling author of *Hashimoto's Thyroiditis*

"An empowering guide filled with keen insight and heartfelt compassion that can help every woman or man feel beautiful inside and out."
—Michael T. Murray, N.D., co-author of *The Encyclopedia of Natural Medicine*

"*Clean Skin from Within* shines with insightful information for anyone wanting to look and feel their youthful best from the inside out."
—Razi Berry, publisher, *Naturopathic Doctor News & Review* and *NaturalPath*

"Finally, a plan for healthy skin that zeroes in on the real and lasting solution!"
—Lise Alschuler, N.D., F.A.B.N.O., co-author of *Definitive Guide to Cancer* and *Definitive Guide to Thriving After Cancer*

"You can get your natural radiance and confidence back, and this book will show you how."
—Cynthia Pasquella, celebrity nutritionist, best-selling author, and host of *What You're Really Hungry For*

Dr. Trevor Cates
The Spa Dr.
TheSpaDr.com/specialoffer

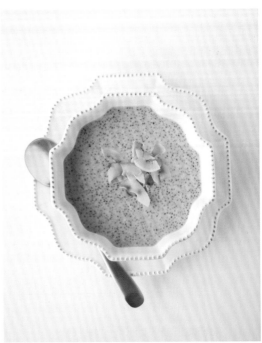
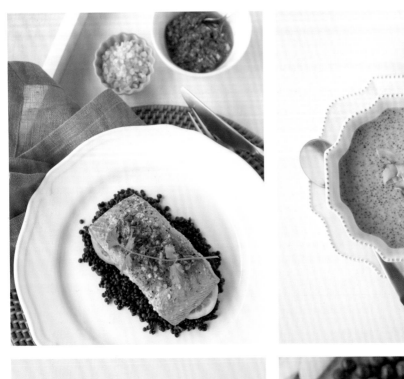
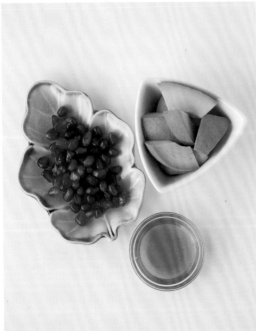
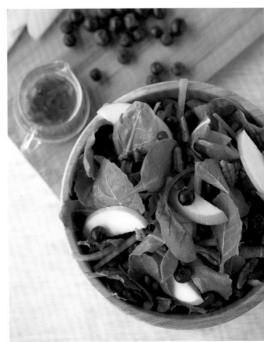

CONTENTS

Foreword

"Beauty is more than skin deep" is far more than an adage. What we apply to our skin has a potentially tremendous impact on our health, and the health of our skin is a reflection of much deeper processes happening in our bodies.

Absorbed through the deeper layers of our skin, the personal care products we apply on the surface find their way into our cells. Even tiny amounts of certain ingredients can act as cancer-causing carcinogens, obesogens that bind with hormonal and fat cells to activate obesity genes, and endocrine disruptors. The latter chemicals behave as estrogen and testosterone in our body, causing hormonal imbalances that can lead to a host of problems, including early puberty in young girls, acne, infertility, thyroid disorders, menstrual problems, polycystic ovarian syndrome (PCOS), weight issues, and diabetes.

What we put on our skin should be as clean as what we eat. But for most people, it's not. By the time we walk out the door in the morning, most of us, both men and women, have applied as many as fifteen different skin and hair products, with at least 126 unique ingredients. Even in tiny amounts, many of the chemicals commonly found in our cosmetics can have a tremendous health and hormonal impact, and we are only beginning to understand the consequences of how they interact on our skin and in our detoxification systems.

In my Integrative and Functional Medicine practice, I have identified high levels of chemicals that come from cosmetics in the blood of patients struggling with hormonal, weight, skin, and even mood troubles. The scary part is that most of the ingredients we apply to our skin are not regulated the same way foods and medications do, leaving our bodies to be the lab benches on which science experiments are conducted. So far, the results are troubling. As a culture, we're experiencing unprecedented rates of skin problems, hormonal imbalances, autoimmune disease, depression, obesity, diabetes, and dementia—all of which can be associated with harmful, system-disrupting chemical exposures.

Yet many of us apply this tremendous number of lotions and cosmetics to cover skin blemishes and give us the glow that our hurried, stressed lives seem to keep us from having naturally. And we're trying to keep up with unrealistic beauty norms. Having been in front of the camera on television and for magazines, I know that it takes enormous amounts of makeup, continually reapplied, to look like a cover model. But that is not truly clear, glowing skin; it is an illusion. However, when I'm rested, eating well, and taking care of myself, I do have glowing, clear, healthy skin—naturally.

I share the philosophy that Dr. Trevor Cates so beautifully presents to you in this scientifically sound and visually delightful book: that the health of our skin is a reflection of the health of deeper processes in our body. These include our gut health, detoxification systems, hormonal balance, stress levels, and nutritional status, all of which affect what happens on the surface. Or more simply put: Clean skin starts from within.

I have known Dr. Cates for the past three years and have come to admire her for her commitment to taking scientific research and making it practical; her high standards as a practitioner; and also for the ingredients she uses to formulate her skin care products. As Dr. Cates says, "skin is our magic mirror," and, in my own practice, I see this in patients when their acne or eczema flares up after a weekend sugar binge, a "night out with the girls" and a bit of drinking, or during times of high stress and overwork (which is a lot of the time for most of us). I see a positive change in skin radiance when missing nutrients are incorporated by way of diet or, if needed, supplements; when liver function is supported by the right nutrients; and when digestion is cleared up. Struggling with severe acne, sensitive skin, or reactions like eczema and hives can have a big emotional impact. When you learn to adjust your diet and lifestyle, and begin to nourish yourself from within, your skin clears up and the relief is profound.

Yet I can tell you, as a Yale University-trained medical doctor, this is not something your doctor learned in medical school. And that's why this book is so important. We've been chasing the appearance of health and beauty with cosmetics, and even potentially dangerous pharmaceuticals, when beauty truly is more than skin deep. In my philosophy, healthy is the new beauty. And we can't get healthy using unhealthy ingredients.

In my practice and personal life, as you will find in Dr. Cates's book as well, a natural approach using fresh, nutrient-rich foods and skin care products made with ingredients that are just as fresh and natural is the golden ticket. The great news is that your body really knows what to do when given the right tools and support—and Dr. Cates's two-week plan provides the blueprint. This program is a great way to reset your health and habits for a lifetime of healthy skin and optimal health.

Having a beauty routine is arguably something I wasn't doing enough of, as my three daughters would tell you. Despite being well known in the health and wellness world, being a busy mom with four kids and a professional life, I splashed water on my face in the morning, did the same in the evening, and in the summers used an organic sunscreen if I planned to get heavy sun exposure. I considered skin care a luxury that I had no time for. Fortunately, decent genes, avoiding harmful body products, an excellent diet, and a natural lifestyle kept my skin healthy enough. But when, at the urging of my twenty-two-year old daughter, who began doing research on how French women care for their skin (daily with a less-is-more attitude) and with a gift from Dr. Cates of her skin care products, I began a gentle beauty care routine. I discovered how wrong I was in considering this time to care for myself an unnecessary luxury. A beauty routine is not self-indulgence, it is self-preservation, self-love, and self-care. And you deserve that. Dr. Cates lays the healthiest path for you—and it's right at your fingertips in this book. Enjoy the glow.

—AVIVA ROMM, M.D.

Author of *The Adrenal Thyroid Revolution* and *Botanical Medicines for Women's Health*, winner of the American Botanical Council's James A. Duke Excellence in Botanical Literature Award

The Spa Doctor—How I'm Different from a Dermatologist

When it comes to health and skin, I've been through a lot, learned along the way, and promise to share with you how to look and feel your best at any age. In this book my goal is to help you discover graceful aging and natural beauty using my two-week program for clean, glowing skin and vibrant health.

MY PERSONAL EXPERIENCE

Most of us, at some point, have seen a dermatologist or other health care provider who filled a prescription for a topical or oral medication for skin woes, such as acne, rashes, bumps, or wrinkles. Maybe the prescription worked; maybe it didn't. The thing most people in this scenario have in common is their dermatologist's tendency to look at skin problems through a singular lens—and directly suppress the symptom in question at first glance. While common, the issue with that approach is that merely suppressing symptoms doesn't address the root cause of the problem.

I have personal experience with this type of treatment and can attest to how frustrating it can be. I've always had finicky skin. Hives and eczema during childhood, acne as a teenager, and rosacea in my thirties—you name it and I've probably had it.

Like most children, I wasn't that concerned with how I looked, but the frustration I'd feel after spontaneously breaking out in hives, or seeing a mosquito bite swell to three times its size, was still palpable. Yet, as any caring parents would do, mine took me to every type of specialist imaginable. All prescribed antibiotic after antibiotic. When I stopped responding to one drug, they'd just hand me another. All the while, we crossed our fingers in hopes of finding a magic elixir to make all my skin problems vanish.

I remember trying various antihistamines and other allergy drugs that made me either so exhausted I thought I would faint at school—or wound me up to the point I couldn't sleep. As I focused on putting one foot in front of the other, I questioned whether I was alone in my plight. The worst part was I knew I wasn't a "normal" kid, and it showed in my self-esteem. I was bullied at school to the point I had no friends. I was lonely. Now, as a mom of three kids—with my two girls around the age I was when sick and struggling—I hope they never experience what I went through.

I'm thankful my parents didn't lose hope. When they eventually found a holistic practitioner, everything changed. She introduced me to a new medicine I'd never heard of, and was kind, and took time to listen. I felt no other doctor had really listened to me before. After receiving individualized natural medicine, I finally found some relief; as if by magic, my allergic reactions and itchy rashes subsided. Those stubborn symptoms cleared up not because of antibiotics, antihistamines, or steroids but through a more natural approach.

It wasn't until years later, when I attended naturopathic medical school at the National University of Natural Medicine, that I realized I wasn't alone. I discovered many people suffer from skin conditions and seek conventional medical help but do not get their hoped-for results. And then there are those people who don't realize how good their skin can be until they adopt a cleaner, healthier lifestyle. According to the 2010 Global Burden of Disease (GBD) Study, skin conditions are the fourth-leading cause of nonfatal disease burden globally.

For the past seventeen years, I've counseled patients in holistic medicine—helping them adjust their diet, sleep, and exercise routines to aid in weight loss, digestion, and the like. You'd think my personal struggles would compel me to focus solely on natural remedies for skin issues from the get-go. However, it wasn't until about seven years ago, as The Spa Dr. at a world-renowned spa, that an outpouring of patient testimonials prompted me toward this focus.

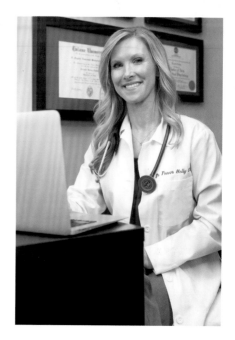

While offering weight-loss advice to hundreds of men and women, many would gush that the lifestyle changes I recommended not only served as a panacea for their primary health concerns but also helped revitalize their complexions. One patient came in with irregular cycles and premenstrual syndrome (PMS). When I addressed her hormone imbalances with dietary advice and detoxification support, she felt better by her next cycle—and, to her pleasant surprise, her acne vanished. Another patient who followed my weight-loss plan lost fifteen pounds and saw the eczema she'd been embarrassed by for years disappear. In these cases, plus countless others, the common bond was addressing the underlying cause of their health woes. The resulting changes, not to mention their newfound confidence, appeared right on the surface of their bodies—their skin!

At that point, the idea that our skin is similar to a magic mirror—offering clues about a person's internal health—really hit home. It's this concept that has guided my practice as The Spa Dr. and served as inspiration for my two-week program for clean, glowing skin and vibrant health. Patients who have tried the program paint the best picture of how daily lifestyle choices have a direct effect on internal health, which, in turn, has a direct effect on the appearance of our skin. In as few as three days, some patients start to find relief for their acne, rosacea, eczema, dry skin, and other common skin conditions. And in two weeks their skin doesn't only begin to clear up—it also starts to glow with a more youthful appearance.

THE STATE OF OUR SKIN

While much of today's conventional treatment is similar to when I was an adolescent struggling with itchy skin and breakouts, the incidence of skin problems and expenses associated with them are growing. The U.S. dermatology market is expected to grow from $10.1 billion to $13.1 billion by 2017. And, according to GBI Research, the global dermatology market is expected to have significant growth, from $20 billion in 2015 to $33.7 billion by 2022. One big reason for the rise in dermatology costs is the aging population. With age comes more skin cancer, as well as concerns about aging—wrinkles, sagging skin, and hyperpigmentation.

Acne is the most common skin condition in the United States—affecting up to 50 million Americans and costing over $3 billion annually. A 2015 review in the *British Journal of Dermatology* reports that acne is estimated to affect 9.4 percent of the world's population, making it the eighth most prevalent disease worldwide.

According to the American Academy of Dermatology, adult-onset acne is on the rise among women in their twenties, thirties, forties, and even fifties—and we're not just talking a few pimples. A 2014 study in the *Journal of Clinical and Aesthetic Dermatology* suggested that in the United States, about 45 percent of women ages twenty-one to thirty had clinical acne, 26 percent of women ages thirty-one to forty had clinical acne, and 12 percent of women ages forty-one to fifty had clinical acne.

Acne sufferers are not alone in their plight. Rosacea is estimated to affect over 16 million Americans. It often appears in women over thirty, as redness, small visible blood vessels, and eruptions on the nose, cheeks, and forehead. Untreated, the problem only gets worse.

An estimated 32 million people have eczema, and at least 17.8 million have moderate to severe eczema or atopic dermatitis, a 2007 study published in *Dermatitis* suggests. Eczema is a broad term that encompasses a few forms of dermatitis. Stress and irritants, such as soaps, allergens, and climate, appear to trigger this condition. Eczema affects children and adults. In adults it often appears on the elbows, on hands, and in skin folds.

Other common skin ailments include psoriasis, dry skin, vitiligo, itchy skin, hives, and infectious skin diseases, including viral conditions such as herpes and warts, fungal skin diseases such as ringworm and athlete's foot, and bacterial skin infections such as impetigo.

And yet, despite the growing number of skin problems people face today, many traditional skin doctors scoff at the idea that what patients eat, and other lifestyle factors, can significantly affect their skin. The American Academy of Dermatology, despite all the research, stated (on February 17, 2016), "There is not enough data to recommend dietary changes for acne patients." Instead, the Academy says, the "recommended treatments include topical therapy, antibiotics, isotretinoin, and oral contraceptives," all of which are palliative but don't support the body's innate ability to heal.

YOU AREN'T ALONE, EITHER

My plan differs from the conventional dermatology approach. I look at undesirable skin symptoms as a sign that something *within* the body is off balance. With my educational training and experience helping thousands of patients, I know the body is a wise entity that, when given the right tools, can reach its full, vibrant potential. In this healthier state, symptoms vanish and there's a greater chance they'll stay at bay. Put differently, when we don't evaluate the body holistically, we can't get to the true underlying cause of skin problems—the body remains inflamed and out of balance, and symptoms reappear in a vicious cycle.

I'm not saying dermatologists don't know skin, nor am I saying the treatments they prescribe don't work. Dermatologists are quite valuable for diagnosing skin conditions and detecting skin cancer, and some research I share in this book on natural treatments comes from forward-thinking dermatologists. Rather, I mean that a holistic approach can get to the root of skin challenges and that subsequent, simple lifestyle and diet changes can significantly alleviate symptoms. I know firsthand that doing so can result in saved money and time—and ultimately in a healthier body and clear, glowing skin.

MY FIVE HOLISTIC SKIN DISCOVERIES

To help us get to the bottom of what's really plaguing your skin, here are five holistic concepts I've discovered about skin.

1. The skin offers a direct reflection of what's happening inside the body.

2. Common prescriptions usually don't fix the true underlying problem.

3. The skin has a delicate pH balance and community of bacteria that are crucial for its health.

4. What you eat can have a big effect on your skin.

5. Products you put on your skin affect internal health.

Let's look at each point.

1. The skin offers a direct reflection of what's happening inside the body.

Our skin is our largest organ, and it provides an outward manifestation of our inner health. When our digestion, hormones, blood sugar, immune system, or other body systems are out of whack, this imbalance often shows up on our skin. If your symptoms are only treated superficially by suppressing them, then you'll miss the opportunity to learn what the body is really trying to tell you.

2. Common prescriptions don't fix the underlying problem.

Most commonly prescribed medications, such as antibiotics and steroids, do not address underlying factors that go beyond what's happening on the skin. Instead they suppress the symptom and can actually worsen a person's health and skin. It's true that we sometimes need antibiotics to treat a bad infection and that steroids can help reduce inflammation. However, these treatments are overused and often used too quickly without first considering more natural options. We know antibiotics zap harmful bacteria, but they also destroy the beneficial bacteria in our bodies at the same time, which can actually worsen the problem in the long run.

3. The skin has a delicate pH balance and community of bacteria that are crucial for its health.

As the wealth of knowledge from research continues to grow, we're learning more about the benefits of bugs within our digestive system and also on our skin. One key finding is the role of the *gut microbiome*. The human digestive tract contains a delicate balance of microorganisms, including bacteria. A well-functioning digestive tract has the right amount of good bugs (such as lactobacillus) but not bad bugs (such as harmful bacteria, parasites, or an overgrowth of candida). Throughout our lives, when we encounter toxins, stress, infections, poor dietary choices, antibiotics, and other medications, our precious microbiome is compromised; so, in turn, is the health of our skin.

Our skin has its own microbiome that helps keep it clear of blemishes and breakouts—and prevents premature aging. When skin lotions and treatments disturb our skin's delicate pH balance, our skin microbiome is affected. While trying to treat the issues, we're only making it worse when we disrupt the pH and microbiome!

4. What you eat can have a big effect on your skin.

An increasing amount of research has emerged that absolutely debunks doctors who deny that what we eat affects skin quality. For example, a 2014 study in the *Journal of Drugs in Dermatology* suggests eating foods with a high glycemic index (GI), such as refined carbohydrates, plays a role in the development of acne. Research published in 2008 in the *Journal of the American Academy of Dermatology* also suggests skim milk can trigger acne.

On the other hand, many nutrients and foods can and do nourish skin from the inside out. For example, consuming omega-3 fatty acids and gamma linolenic acids (GLAs) may help reduce acne breakouts, suggests a 2014 study published in the international journal *Acta Dermato-Venereologica*.

5. Products you put on your skin affect internal health.

Did you know that many skin care products contain endocrine-disrupting chemicals (EDCs) and that some are even carcinogenic? EDCs are a problem because they interfere with our hormone function. Although you may think that something you apply to your skin stays only on your skin, the chemicals in our skin care products can actually be absorbed into our bloodstream. These chemicals can then wreak havoc on our endocrine system, leading to problems with thyroid, adrenal, and sex hormone function. According to the Endocrine Society, a research and advocacy group focused on hormones and endocrinology, EDCs are associated with fertility issues, breast development, breast cancer, prostate cancer, thyroid disease, neuroendocrine problems, obesity, and cardiovascular disease. In a 2009 study published in its journal, *Endocrine Reviews*, the Endocrine Society described EDCs as "a significant concern to public health." One important step for reducing exposure to EDCs is to look more carefully at what you put on your skin.

POTENTIAL PROBLEMS WITH TYPICAL DERMATOLOGY PRESCRIPTIONS

Antibiotics are one of the most common treatments for skin problems such as acne. As a result, we're now seeing more bacteria resistance—even zits that are antibiotic resistant. While eliminating harmful bacteria, antibiotics also kill the "good" bacteria that enhance our digestion and protect our skin.

Topical corticosteroids are another popular dermatologists' prescription to treat eczema, psoriasis, and itchy rashes. Corticosteroids work by suppressing the immune system, which reduces inflammation and associated itching. There are various forms and strengths of topical steroids that are intended for short-term use. The potential side effects include infection, thinning skin, hyperpigmentation, and irritation. But the real problem is that you're covering up rather than addressing the underlying cause of what triggered your skin condition. Dermatologists usually stick with topical steroids, but sometimes physicians will prescribe oral corticosteroids, which have uncommon but more serious potential side effects such as Cushing disease, high blood sugar, and HPA axis suppression (hypothalamus-pituitary-adrenal suppression, which creates an imbalance by suppressing the function of these three endocrine glands).

Although less common today, topical coal tar is another conventional treatment for itchy, scaly, flaky skin, such as from psoriasis, eczema, and seborrheic dermatitis. The shampoos, lotions, creams, gels, ointments, scalp treatments, and other products are available both in over-the-counter (OTC) and prescription forms. The problem is that coal tar is derived from coal, a known carcinogen, according to the education and advocacy group Campaign for Safe Cosmetics.

A 2012 National Health Statistics report published by the Centers for Disease Control and Prevention (CDC) estimated that more than 60 percent of women of reproductive age use contraception—and nearly 30 percent of those women are on the pill. Although the American Academy of

Pediatrics recommends using the pill to help prevent unintended pregnancy, doctors often prescribe hormonal contraceptives to alleviate acne. But some birth control pills can worsen a woman's health by throwing hormones, including cortisol and testosterone, off balance, as well as leading to nutritional deficiencies.

Accutane was used to treat acne in 5 million Americans before the company's prescription drug unit, Hoffmann-La Roche, discontinued its U.S. sales in 2009 amid concerns of side effects such as suicidal behavior, psychosis, miscarriages, and birth deformities. But the same drug—generically known as isotretinoin—is still on the market and sold under alternative names, including Absorica, Amnesteem, Claravis, Myorisan, and Zenatane. While isotretinoin is known to help clear up severe acne that is resistant to other treatments, there are still concerns about serious potential side effects, including major birth defects, depression, suicidal thoughts, liver toxicity, dry skin, high cholesterol, and inflammatory bowel disease. Some non-pregnant consumers may decide with their dermatologist that their wish to relieve acne outweighs these potential health risks. However, it is important to understand that there are alternatives to try first before resorting to isotretinoin.

In some cases, skin conditions are so extreme that a combination approach might be useful. In these cases, such as severe acne, conventional medications can be used to calm the inflammation to a more manageable place so that natural therapies can provide the healing. I realize conventional medicine can help manage symptoms, but my concern is that many dermatology treatments are overused or used without supporting the body's innate ability to heal. If you do choose to go down the road of these medications, make sure you closely follow your doctor's instructions to help avoid unwanted side effects.

DISCOVERING A HEALTHIER SKIN REGIMEN

Despite the influx of new drugs and their claims as one-stop shops and silver-bullet remedies, skin complications aren't subsiding—they're multiplying. In 2013 global beauty and personal care was worth $454 billion—a number that is expected to grow, according to Euromonitor International data. It's no wonder these products, not to mention aesthetic procedures such as BOTOX Cosmetic injections and plastic surgery, are so popular. They promise miraculous results without calling for lifestyle changes, which, as any of my patients who've followed my two-week plan will tell you, is a tragic oversight.

Look, I get it. I'm in my forties, and I realize having radiant skin doesn't get any easier with age. Wrinkles aren't all that bad—they're signs we've been living and laughing. The most beautiful women I've ever known have been in their seventies and eighties. But I know none of us want to look older than we are. While we may have to work a little harder, I have learned it is still possible to have clear, glowing skin as we age. Both skin care and diet play a big role in healthy aging.

The good news is that in just two weeks, with my program for glowing skin and vibrant health, patients with skin care woes from eczema to psoriasis and acne to aging usually see their symptoms improve.

Back when I was first practicing in spas and started to see more and more patients with skin issues, they asked me which skin care products they should use. I counseled them about EDCs and toxins in popular skin care products, and so they wanted to know which were safe. I explained my focus was healthy skin from *within* . . . but my patients kept asking.

My estheticians and dermatologist friends told me, "Natural skin care products are okay, but they just don't work. You'll have to choose between natural *or* effective."

I wasn't happy with that answer, so I decided to do more research. That research led me to the science of natural beauty and to create my own line of skin care products— The Spa Dr.—designed to be clean, natural, *and effective*.

Whether you choose my skin care line, make your own products (as in chapter 9), or opt for other high-quality natural skin care options, external nourishment is just as important as internal nourishment for clear, youthful-looking skin.

As for that little girl who suffered through many a skin woe, I am much more confident now. You could argue that empowering others and relating to their desire to achieve a healthy complexion has played a role, and you'd be right. But I believe my commitment to practicing what I preach has something to do with it, too.

Berfore you read on to explore this two-week program, it will be helpful to figure out your skin type. Go to TheSkinQuiz.com to take my easy skin quiz and get the most out of this book.

> *"The good news is that in just two weeks, with my program for glowing skin and vibrant health, patients with skin care woes from eczema to psoriasis and acne to aging usually see their symptoms improve."*

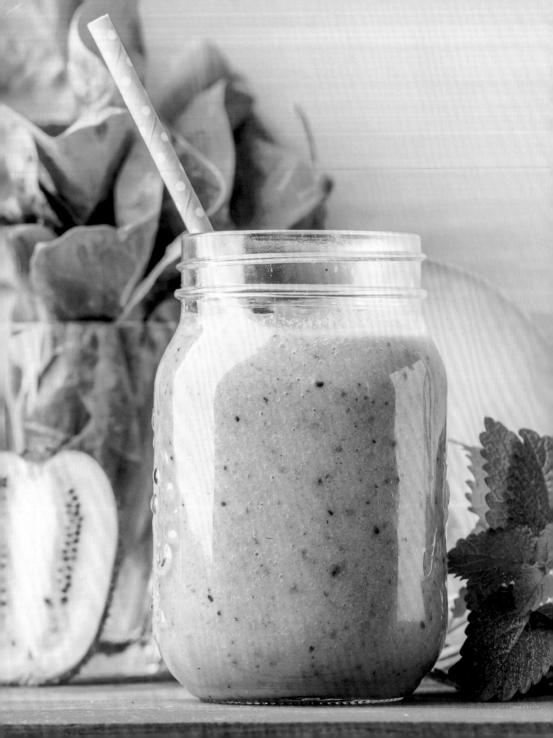

PART ONE

A DIFFERENT APPROACH TO SKIN

Tracy, a thirty-six-year-old real estate agent, arrived at my office with a beautiful complexion veiled by acne, as well as an armful of skin care products for which she had dished out hundreds of dollars. I remember her frustration vividly: "I'm so tired of trying all these things and not getting anywhere," she said. "I still feel like a teenager." Tracy explained she also had, per her physician's advice, experimented with various birth control pills, antibiotics, and steroid creams—only to be left fed up and with no results.

I assured Tracy this time would be different—that I wasn't like traditional dermatologists—and shared my approach with her. In just two weeks she returned to my office with clearer skin and a brighter outlook on life.

"Now I see why my friend told me I had to see just one more doctor," she gushed, "you."

While you can't assess the health of your liver, kidneys, heart, or other organs without technology that allows you to peer into the body, it's easy to see the organ most representative of your overall health without assistance: the skin. While that reality may make you feel exposed, it's actually fortunate. Think of it this way: Your skin is like a magic mirror—a device that can offer clues about how healthy your habits are and what's happening to your body's internal systems. When we look at what's happening on the surface of our skin and understand the causes behind those symptoms, it's easier to make daily changes to improve how we look and feel. Let's delve deeper into that.

CHAPTER 1

Your Magic Mirror and Its Clues

When you look at your skin in the bathroom mirror, what do you see? If your skin is imperfect (Whose isn't?), your first instinct may be to mask any redness, bumps, fine lines, and discolorations with foundation, powder, or a similar concealing makeup. But have you ever stopped and really thought about why your skin contains blemishes in the first place? Checking for the hints your skin gives you to figure out the "why" is what this magic-mirror concept is all about.

Let's back up and discuss what *healthy* skin looks like. If you look at any healthy baby, you'll see a quality of skin similar to the kind you once had—before the weather, the sun, and various lifestyle choices took their tolls. I'm not saying we all *need* completely flawless skin—as the saying goes, there's no such thing as perfect—but the fact is, when your skin isn't healthy, neither is the rest of your body. Ultimately, achieving overall health, inside and out, is something we can all agree is a good thing. That's the goal here.

Now let's try this exercise: Take a close look at your face in the mirror. If you have one of those mirrors that magnifies, even better.

Do you see any of the following: Redness, discoloration, bumps, blood vessels, dryness, enlarged pores, whiteheads, blackheads, freckles, areas of excess pigmentation or lack of pigmentation, cracks (in the corners of your mouth), wrinkles, or sagging skin?

Make a note if you do.

Do the symptoms change from day to day, week to week, month to month, or do they appear sporadically? Those are important variables to consider, and they're worth recording because they will help you tailor your skin care routine based on my recommendations in this book.

Now, take a deep breath. Remember: You're beautiful and you shouldn't let any perceived skin flaws bring you down. They're simply a signal that something else is out of balance within your body. With the proper assistance we can kick our bodies' natural healing functions into gear to help resolve those issues. First, though, we need to do some detective work to understand how your magic mirror can lead you to the ultimate remedy that's best for you.

THE SIX CAUSES BEHIND IMPERFECT SKIN

There are six main underlying causes that can lead to imperfect skin:

1. Inflammation

2. Microbiome disturbance

3. Oxidative damage

4. Blood sugar issues

5. Nutritional deficiencies

6. Hormonal imbalances

You probably won't hear your traditional dermatologist talk about these six factors. But I can tell you with confidence, based on my experience and the results I've seen with my patients, that investigating how these elements may be affecting your body can help solve the mystery behind your skin qualms.

The idea is that if we can identify the underlying cause, we'll then find the weak spot that can lead to the most common skin problems, such as acne, eczema, rosacea, and premature aging. When you address your specific Achilles heel, coming up with treatment tailored just for you is much easier.

Many of these root causes are related to genetics, but the good news is you're not stuck with bad outcomes just because of the hand you're dealt at birth. You can, through a healthy diet, lifestyle, and natural medicine, positively change your genetic expression.

Let's explore these six causes of imperfect skin. Then we'll delve into the skin types commonly associated with each so you can connect the dots and learn how to identify (and treat) your underlying issues.

CAUSE #1: INFLAMMATION

Inflammation can have enormous effec the body, including the skin. "Skinflam tion," as I call it, can make skin more ser tive and can cause you to be more susceptible to eczema, dermatitis, psoriasis, acne, rosacea, and most chronic skin conditions.

Externally, when skin is triggered by exposure to UV radiation, allergens, or irritating soaps or cosmetics, skin cells produce cytokines and chemokines—inflammatory hormones that bind to certain cell receptors and then trigger more inflammatory hormones. This leads to increased blood flow (vasodilation), and may trigger immune cells to travel to the skin to add to the body's inflammatory response.

Similarly, an inflammatory response occurs internally with anything the immune system deems a threat, such as viruses, toxins, food allergens or intolerances, and, in some cases, medications. When something enters the body that the immune system detects as foreign, such as bacteria viruses, histamine—which is made and stored within our white blood cells—acts as an inflammatory mediator. This is one of the internal changes that occur in the immune system and lead to inflammation. When inflammation occurs, the body feels under attack and responds accordingly, and one place this phenomenon presents itself is on the skin.

Skinflammation problems often stem from digestive issues. Related to the delicate balance of our gut microflora is the dreaded "leaky gut." Our digestive tract has a somewhat permeable lining, but when that lining becomes more permeable than it should be, food particles can slip through. Our immune system sees those particles as foreign substances. This creates an inflammatory response in the body, and one of the main effects we see is skin disturbance, which can take the form of eczema, acne, or a number of other skin ailments.

CAUSE #2: MICROBIOME DISTURBANCE

The human digestive tract contains a delicate balance of microorganisms called the *gut microbiome*. Friendly bacteria (such as lactobacillus and bifidobacteria) help crowd out harmful bacteria, parasites, or overgrowth of candida. Exposure to our mothers' flora during birth typically sets us up for a healthy gut microbiome. But as we age, toxins, stress, infections, poor dietary choices, and certain medications can negatively affect the gut microbiome (leading to inflammation, among other things).

The gut's health is directly related to our skin's health. A healthy gut microbiome protects the gut lining, increases the body's ability to absorb nutrients, and protects against harmful microorganisms that affect healthy skin. A well-balanced gut microbiome will help keep your skin clear and glowing.

In addition to your gut microbiome, the body also has a skin microbiome that contains different yet equally important microorganisms living on, and protecting, this organ. A well-balanced skin microbiome protects your skin from harmful pathogens and promotes the natural lipid barrier and skin immune system. Ultimately this function helps prevent acne, eczema, other blemishes, and premature aging, which can take the form of excess wrinkles and sagging skin. For example, good bugs on your skin prevent harmful bacteria overgrowth, such as *Propionibacterium acnes*, which is believed to be a major trigger for acne.

Research suggests that probiotics, or good bacteria, have helped remedy various skin conditions. These have been used successfully both topically on skin and orally. More on that later. For now, know that a healthy microbiome is important internally (in your gut) as well as externally (on your skin), and an unhealthy one may be the culprit behind a variety of skin issues.

CAUSE #3: OXIDATIVE DAMAGE

Because skin acts as an external barrier, it is directly exposed to environmental stress, such as sunlight and pollutants. Excessive exposure to the sun's UV radiation generates free radicals in the skin, and when their levels exceed the organ's natural antioxidant defenses, oxidative damage occurs. That effect can present as premature aging, sunburn, skin inflammation, and skin cancers. It also causes depletion of antioxidants, such as vitamins E and C, which further reduces their protective effects.

Aging itself is a form of oxidative stress because antioxidant levels in the skin and blood reduce as we age and we lose that built-in protection. Because oxidative damage can lead to genetic mutations and telomere shortening (stretches of DNA at the ends of chromosomes that protect our genetic data, which shorten each time a cell divides until they can no longer divide and die)—all associated with accelerated aging—it can make us look and feel older than we are. Free radicals damage collagen and affect the firmness and suppleness of our skin, leading to dryness, fine lines, and wrinkles, as well as less elasticity—and that's just skimming the surface.

Oxidative damage occurs externally from sun and pollutants, but it also occurs internally from toxins and poor dietary choices. This extends to internal organs as well, and even increases our risk of developing chronic diseases. We know, however, that certain lifestyle choices and natural medicine can help combat these effects.

CAUSE #4: BLOOD SUGAR ISSUES

The body uses glucose (blood sugar) as a primary fuel source, but if glucose is consumed in excess, or not used and metabolized properly, it can bind to skin's collagen and elastin, which can damage skin. This process is called glycation, and its end products, called advanced glycation end products (AGEs), cause our skin to become rigid and less elastic. The end result: cracked, thin, and red skin with a weakened ability to repair itself that is prone to wrinkles and accelerated aging. Research suggests that once the cross-linking of glucose with collagen and elastin occurs, it is hard to reverse.

Just how fast glycation occurs is partially genetic, but lifestyle choices can play a role. Consuming sugar, or anything that turns to sugar in the body, increases blood glucose and is the major contributor to glycation. Other foods, depending on the method of preparation, may contain preformed AGEs. High-heat cooking methods, such as barbecuing, grilling, frying, and roasting, lead to higher levels of AGEs. It has been shown that adding acidic ingredients, such as lemon juice or vinegar, can help reduce AGEs.

In addition to the aging effects of glycation, when blood sugar rises so does insulin, which can increase sebum production and lead to acne breakouts. In other pathways, high blood sugar and glycation lead to inflammation, which can trigger a host of additional skin concerns.

"The gut's health is directly related to our skin's health."

CAUSE #5: NUTRITIONAL DEFICIENCIES

Some of the first signs of nutritional deficiencies appear on our skin. These can be from micronutrient deficiencies (vitamins and minerals) as well as macronutrient deficiencies (carbohydrates, fats, and protein). Nutritional deficiencies are most common in people with restrictive or inadequate nutrient diets, excessive consumption of alcohol, or digestion and absorption issues. However, I've seen patients who appear to be living a relatively healthy lifestyle yet still have nutritional deficiencies. So it's good to be proactive and ensure that you're properly nourished, which we'll discuss at length in the chapters ahead.

SOME SYMPTOMS OF VITAMIN DEFICIENCIES

Iron and B vitamin deficiencies (especially vitamins B_2 and B_{12}) can cause painful cracks, blisters, or crusting in the corners of your mouth (called *angular cheilitis*, or *cheilosis*). This is more common than you might think; luckily it's easy to treat. I developed this during medical school when I was under a lot of stress and not making healthy food choices, but the condition vanished as soon as I had a B vitamin injection.

Another common skin issue linked to vitamin deficiency can appear in the form of small white or red bumps on the backs of your arms, cheeks, buttocks, or thighs called *keratosis pilaris*. These look like tiny pimples, and they usually occur when you're not getting enough essential fatty acids, zinc, or vitamin A in your diet. Run your fingers across the backs of your upper arms to check for any tiny bumps or rough skin.

People also experience rough skin when the skin is dry. Chronic dry skin and dandruff is often the result of an essential fatty acid deficiency. There is a reason these fatty acids, such as omega-3s, are called "essential"—we need them!

While cheilosis, keratosis pilaris, chronic dry skin, and dandruff are relatively common, some conditions resulting from a vitamin deficiency are less prevalent today but result in more severe symptoms. For example, a significant vitamin C deficiency can cause scurvy or reddish-bluish bruise-like spots surrounding hair follicles, usually on the shins (perifollicular papules and hyperkeratotic plaques). Fortunately, decreasing your risk of suffering from this problem is simple: Consume at least 30 to 60 mg of vitamin C daily—or about a half cup (120 ml) of freshly squeezed orange juice. Knowing how skin ailments are linked to vitamin deficiencies is a crucial first step to achieving a glowing complexion.

CAUSE #6: HORMONAL IMBALANCES

When our hormones are off balance, we are more likely to develop skin problems such as dry skin, fine lines and wrinkles, acne, or rosacea—and sometimes more than one of these blights at the same time. Hormones are biochemical messengers used by the endocrine system to communicate with itself and the rest of the body's systems. Hormones are derived from amino acids, phospholipids, and cholesterol, and they play a significant role in many aspects of our health.

Just how much they rule our physiology may surprise you. From our mental focus, memory, and cognition to sex drive, cardiovascular health, bone growth, sugar regulation, and metabolism, hormones play a major role in our bodies, and imbalance is one major underlying cause of health problems. Hormones also have a symbiotic relationship with one another, which means if one hormone is out of balance, there's a domino effect. That one imbalance affects the normal signals to hormones and either decreases or increases other hormone levels.

Many hormones play a role in the health of your skin—from adrenal (cortisol and DHEA) and thyroid to melatonin (our sleep hormone) and sex hormones (estrogen, progesterone, and testosterone). Melatonin and DHEA, for example, are both found in human skin and have protective functions.

While some hormones help protect our skin from blemishes and aging, others can promote those symptoms. For example, when elevated, the stress hormone cortisol triggers inflammation, which can exacerbate skin problems. Cortisol is not all bad. We need it to help us wake up in the morning and be alert throughout the day.

As with many things in life, it's really about balance. All of our hormones play an important role in our health, but when they're out of balance, problems occur.

PUTTING IT ALL TOGETHER

At this point you're probably wondering which root causes apply to you. There's a good chance more than one (or maybe all) of these factors are holding you back from clear, glowing skin. To help identify your primary weak spots, I've defined five classic skin types, each of which is connected to a specific combination of the six underlying causes.

Traditionally, skin types are divided into categories such as dry, oily, combination, and sensitive. I believe there are more layers, and that this categorization does not help an individual address the *underlying causes* of skin qualms. That's why I've redefined those types. If you see a dermatologist or esthetician, this approach is likely different from what they've discussed with you, but I think you'll find it makes sense and provides clear solutions.

THE SPA DR.'S
FIVE SKIN TYPES

I look at patients as people rather than objects that exhibit the skin condition at hand. So I have given each type a human name rather than labeling each as a disease. Many conventional doctors put patients into boxes—"forty-six-year-old female with psoriasis," for example—and then prescribe whatever treatment they think will help. That approach doesn't take the whole picture into account, so it doesn't unveil the root cause.

Keeping in mind that whatever ails your skin doesn't define you, as you read these descriptions inspired by some of my patients,

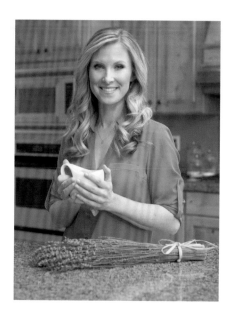

you will likely find one you can relate to. It's very likely you will relate to more than one or two. Note which one(s) sounds like you. Later, I'll explain how to address the underlying causes associated with each type so that you can address your specific issues.

AMBER

Amber, a thirty-seven-year-old stay-at-home mom of two, came to me at her wit's end struggling with dark pigmentation along her cheeks. She tried to conceal the discoloration and even out her skin tone with makeup, but her efforts proved futile; her splotchy skin continued to make her self-conscious and look older than her age. She used skin-lightening lotions, only to discover that her skin was then increasingly prone to more darkened areas. To top it off, she tried hydroquinone, to which she had an allergic

Key features of the "Amber" skin type

▸ Hyperpigmentation (darkening of skin in certain areas)

▸ Freckles

▸ Melasma (brown or gray-brown patches that usually appear on the cheeks, bridge of the nose, forehead, or upper lip); also called the "mask of pregnancy" but can plague individuals who are not pregnant

▸ Uneven skin tone

reaction. She told me, "I just can't get rid of this! It keeps getting worse and worse. I'm so embarrassed."

If you're like Amber, after going in the sun, your skin pigments appear in certain areas in the form of freckles or melasma. Sunscreen helps prevent additional pigmentation, but once these characteristics appear, they usually linger. You could conceal them with makeup, but you may feel splotchy and self-conscious. If you've been pregnant or taken birth control pills, you may have noticed that the pigmentation worsens during that time.

You may have tried skin-lightening creams and treatments, meaning you have to be extra cautious in the sun because you're even more prone to hyperpigmentation. The popular lightening treatment for Amber-type hyperpigmentation is hydroquinone, but studies have reported allergenic and carcinogenic properties, so look for healthier alternatives, such as turmeric.

For the Amber skin type, there are two underlying root causes at play: *oxidative damage* and *hormone imbalance*.

ROOT CAUSE #1: OXIDATIVE DAMAGE

In general we want to prevent pigmentation changes to skin because they're signs of sun damage, and they can also signal internal disturbances. Our skin is our outer protective layer that is susceptible to external influences, such as sun and pollutants. To explain this further, here's a brief anatomy/physiology lesson.

Our epidermis is the top layer of skin and is very thin. The flat cells of the upper layer are called *squamous cells*; below this are *basal cells. Melanocytes* are cells that also reside in the epidermis. These cells make the brown pigment melanin, which gives skin its tan or brown color and helps protect against damaging effects of UV rays. Increased melanin production is what leads to hyperpigmentation. The excess production is thought to be caused by sun exposure, inflammation, free radicals, and hormonal changes.

When we experience oxidative stress from sun exposure, oxidative damage occurs. This spirals into increased melanin production to protect the skin and thus worsens hyperpigmentation. If oxidative damage persists, cancer can develop in these various cells, which can mutate, possibly resulting in squamous cell cancer, basal cell cancer, or melanoma.

ROOT CAUSE #2: HORMONAL IMBALANCE

Amber-types are affected by the stress hormone cortisol. This adrenal hormone increases when we're stressed and triggers inflammatory pathways in the body. Because inflammation and oxidative damage work hand in hand to damage skin, this process can worsen hyperpigmentation.

Melasma is often triggered by pregnancy, birth control pills, and hormone therapy. Changes in the hormones estrogen and progesterone cause extra melanin production during sun exposure, leading to melasma.

So we want to balance hormones—both sex hormones (if those are playing a role) and stress hormones.

OLIVIA

Olivia is a forty-three-year-old health coach who came to see me with acne she said was "ruining her life." She shared how the daily breakouts on her face and chest affected her relationship with her husband because she felt the blemishes diminished her attractiveness. The acne also interfered with her ability to do her job well—as a health coach, she didn't feel she offered a good representation of her profession. She tried antibiotics, which helped for a while, but the acne returned with a vengeance when she stopped. For a while she also took birth control pills, but they didn't seem to help. Her dermatologist recommended Accutane, but taking such medications didn't align with her work philosophies. In addition to concerns about the side effects of her prescriptions, the biggest issue was that her problem seemed to worsen over time, not improve.

If you're like Olivia, you tend to have oily skin or easily break out in pimples. It doesn't mean your whole face is oily, but you tend to have at least a few oily areas, such as by your nose or hairline or on your forehead. You've probably tried everything to dry up that excess oil: cleansers, toners, masks, and other topical treatments, perhaps even

Key features of the "Olivia" skin type

- Acne
- Large pores
- Blackheads
- Whiteheads
- Sebaceous hyperplasia (yellowish, soft, small papules on the face, usually on the nose, cheeks, and forehead)

microdermabrasion. Unfortunately, this has likely been doing more harm than good.

Your doctor may have prescribed birth control pills or antibiotics at some point to help address a skin issue. If the issue was really bad, a topical steroid cream or Accutane may have been prescribed. Your skin may have been worse during puberty then started to improve, only to have problems return with a vengeance. Underlying issues at work in this skin type include *blood sugar issues, hormonal imbalance, microbiome disturbance,* and *inflammation.*

ROOT CAUSE #1: BLOOD SUGAR ISSUES

When your blood sugar rises (from dietary or genetic tendencies) insulin production increases, triggering sebum production and androgen activity. All of this leads to those all-too-common yet dreaded acne breakouts. I'm not saying you have to give up sugar forever, but eating a balanced diet while also addressing blood sugar issues will be a great help.

ROOT CAUSE #2: HORMONAL IMBALANCE

In Olivia-type cases, blood sugar is closely related to hormonal imbalance. Insulin is a hormone that helps maintain blood sugar balance. Androgens, such as testosterone, are known to trigger acne. Both men and women have testosterone, and surges during puberty, as well as later in life, can create imbalances. Because cortisol triggers inflammation and acne is inflammatory, you need to balance that as well.

ROOT CAUSE #3: MICROBIOME DISTURBANCE

Gut microbiome health is another trigger for acne in Olivia-types. You're prone to breakouts because of genetics, but when your gut is out of sorts too, acne can rage. In addition to restoring your gut, you need to rebalance your skin microbiome. Once you have acne, your skin microbiome becomes disrupted. Because of this, you'll need to take both an internal and external approach to address the disturbance.

ROOT CAUSE #4: INFLAMMATION

I list this root cause last because the preceding three lead to inflammation. When well balanced, Olivia-types have glowing skin that ages gracefully. But when hormonal imbalances, microbiome disturbances, or blood sugar issues arise, inflammation flares and acne rears its ugly head.

Nutritional deficiencies can play a role here too, but they are not usually the initiator. However, nutrition is key in treating Olivia-types naturally.

HEATH

Heath is a thirty-six-year-old personal trainer who came to see me because he was "fed up" with his red, overly reactive skin. At first he noticed a few small visible blood vessels on his nose. Over time they spread to his

Key features of the "Heath" skin type

▸ Redness or inflammation (maybe even with a bumpy texture)

▸ Easily flushed skin

▸ Sensitive skin (reacts easily to skin care products)

▸ Reaction to weather or temperature

▸ Rosacea (redness on face, cheeks, forehead or chin; may have bumps)

▸ Telangiectasia (visible blood vessels)

cheeks, and then bumps appeared. His dermatologist initially diagnosed the blemishes as acne, but as the redness, inflammation, and bumpy skin worsened, the diagnosis changed to rosacea. He was prescribed antibiotics and creams that either did nothing or inflamed his skin even more. He tried skin care products that further inflamed and dried out his skin. Laser treatments and chemical peels helped at first, but they stopped working after a few months. Heath was beginning to suspect his diet or stress levels were playing a major role in his skin troubles. He shared how the rosacea had been affecting his self-esteem, affecting his work performance, and preventing him from feeling confident enough to date. He was desperate because he read that the condition worsens significantly over time.

If you're like Heath, you have a tendency to have red, inflamed, reactive skin. You may flush more easily than others. If you're a woman, you may try to cover your reddish complexion with makeup. If you have bumps and breakouts, these still show through, and the redness can be annoying and embarrassing. You may have tried creams, topical medications, or antibiotics to squelch the inflammation, or lasers and other light treatments, but your symptoms probably keep returning. According to conventional medicine, there's no cure for rosacea—one key feature of Heath-types—but you can address the root cause, decreasing inflammation naturally and alleviating your skin issues. Factors at work here are *inflammation, microbiome disturbance*, and *hormonal imbalance*.

ROOT CAUSE #1: INFLAMMATION

Inflammation is not your friend when it comes to skin. Redness, swelling, and heat are all signs of external inflammation. These signs of inflammation don't occur only on the outside, however. Most likely you have internal inflammation fueling the fire. When you learn to put out those internal flames, you'll see the skin on your face calm down. When you also eliminate the external inflammation, you'll see the healthy glow you deserve.

ROOT CAUSE #2: MICROBIOME DISTURBANCE

To address inflammation, look at both your internal gut microbiome and your external skin microbiome. Whether a disturbance is the primary trigger or simply contributing to the problem, treating both microbiomes is a great place to start if you're like Heath.

ROOT CAUSE #3: HORMONAL IMBALANCE

Cortisol and other inflammatory hormones are at play here. Balance your inflammatory hormones and you will be that much closer to achieving calm, clear skin.

EMMETT

Emmett is a fifty-two-year-old college professor with itchy, inflamed skin that just "won't go away." Not only did the itching disrupt his sleep, but the patches of skin on his face and torso also made him too embarrassed to take off his shirt at the pool. Little did he know that his affinity for swimming led to excessive chlorine exposure, which in turn made his skin more inflamed. He shared with me that as a child he had a lot of allergies but had "outgrown" them. The skin problems started slowly on his hands and, over eight years, progressively spread to his face, chest, and legs. Emmett tried a prescription steroid topical treatment, as well as various lotions and creams. These somewhat decreased the itching and helped hydrate his skin, but the patches continued to spread. If you're like Emmett, you have chronically dry, scaly skin that may become inflamed and red. Most skin specialists looking at Emmett's list will wonder why I put all of these skin conditions under one category. Because my focus is tackling an underlying cause, I've grouped these characteristics together. These skin issues usually look different from one another, but they all have a root cause in common: an *imbalanced immune system*.

If you're like Emmett, your immune system is either overactive or not performing at its optimal level. You may have been diagnosed with allergies or an autoimmune condition, where the body starts to attack itself. The conventional medical approach has limited treatment options for Emmett-types. You may have tried topical or oral treatments that provided little to no symptom improvement. If you're an Emmett, don't worry: You can experience some relief. Factors at play

Key features of the "Emmett" skin type

- Dry, scaly skin

- Atopic dermatitis (often called eczema, which appears as dry, scaly, and often itchy, red skin)

- Allergic skin reactions, such as hives or contact dermatitis

- Psoriasis (raised reddish or silvery-white scaly patches)

- Keloids (a raised scar that often appears smooth, pink, or purple that can extend beyond the wound site and doesn't improve over time)

- Vitiligo (patches of lighter skin, or depigmentation)

- Seborrheic dermatitis (redness or swelling with a white or yellowish scaling of skin, usually in the center of the face, eyebrows, scalp, and ears)

- Chronic itching

- Recurring acute skin issues and infections (such as impetigo, ringworm, and cold sores)

include *inflammation, microbiome disturbance,* and *hormonal imbalance.*

ROOT CAUSE #1: INFLAMMATION

Immune system overreaction increases inflammatory pathways throughout the body, including the skin. To address inflammation, it's essential for Emmett-types to balance their immune response. This means including anti-inflammatory foods and key

nutrients and avoiding trigger foods that overstimulate your immune system. For additional support, certain immune-balancing herbs and supportive naturopathic treatments can help calm internal and external inflammation.

ROOT CAUSE #2: MICROBIOME DISTURBANCE

Did you know that much of the immune system functions in the gastrointestinal tract? A balanced gut microbiome can help support a healthy immune response. Taking probiotics can help address imbalances and hyperpermeability of your gut, which triggers immune system overactivity.

When your skin microbiome shows signs of being compromised—dry skin, itching, or any chronic skin problem listed previously— you'll want to boost the good microorganisms on your skin too. This will help restore your skin to a smooth, healthy glow.

ROOT CAUSE #3: HORMONAL IMBALANCE

Hormonal imbalances fuel the inflammation and immune reactivity of Emmett-types. If you are an Emmett, like Olivia or Heath, this root cause will be important to address.

SAGE

Sage is a fifty-two-year-old teacher who came to see me because she felt she'd been aging rapidly since turning fifty. Compared to her girlfriends, she felt she had more wrinkles and sagging skin. She asked her closest friends if they'd had plastic surgery but, to her surprise, they had not. Thinking back, she realized her mother and sisters had also gone through abrupt physical changes in their forties and fifties. She wondered if all

Key features of the "Sage" skin type

▸ Sagging skin

▸ Loose skin

▸ Excessive wrinkles

▸ Chronic dry skin

▸ Delayed wound healing

▸ Thin skin

the years as a lifeguard in her twenties or as a nature guide in her thirties had damaged her skin. She was angry with herself for not wearing more sunscreen but noted, "Tans were popular then!" She was thinking about a facelift despite her objections to them in the past. She wanted to age gracefully but felt she was running out of solutions.

If you're a Sage, you are probably more than forty years old and feel you're aging more rapidly than your friends. It's normal for our skin to change as we age because collagen and elastin wear down with time, as well as with greater exposure to weather elements and certain lifestyle factors. Still, we all want to look our age or younger. Luckily, natural remedies that don't require a visit to the plastic surgeon or the purchase of pricey makeup products can help you do just that.

As a Sage-type, you likely have genes passed on from your parents that make you more susceptible to premature or excessive collagen loss. The good news is that we can change our genetic expression by modifying our lifestyle. Genetics and collagen loss play a big role in forming the quality of Sage-type skin, but fortunately we can make significant improvements on those

fronts by addressing the other root causes that affect genetic expression and collagen. They are *oxidative damage, blood sugar issues, hormonal imbalances*, and *nutritional deficiencies*.

ROOT CAUSE #1: OXIDATIVE DAMAGE

Oxidative damage speeds the breakdown of your skin's elastin and collagen. As we age, elastin fibers in skin deteriorate, causing a loss in elasticity, or what keeps your skin wrinkle free. Collagen comprises 70 to 80 percent of skin's dry weight and gives the dermis its structure. Elastin is a relatively small part of the dermis, but its function is important. With age, collagen production gradually declines, and our skin becomes thinner.

In certain hereditary disorders, collagen or elastin is deficient, which leads to accelerated aging. Sun exposure—especially ultraviolet radiation—also causes skin to lose elasticity and age quickly. Usually, the biggest changes occur after age sixty, but with excessive sun exposure, changes can occur as early as our twenties.

You can't stop the clock, but you can reduce oxidative damage through certain dietary and lifestyle changes.

ROOT CAUSE #2: BLOOD SUGAR ISSUES

As I mentioned before, glycation (from excess sugar intake) makes collagen lose its structure, which then makes skin more prone to wrinkles and sagging. Because of any genetic predisposition you may have, pay particular attention to your blood sugar. I'm not saying you can never eat sweets. Rather, it's time to keep an eye on your consumption and support healthy blood sugar balance through some simple diet and lifestyle changes.

ROOT CAUSE #3: HORMONAL IMBALANCES

As we age, our hormones change significantly. While most of our hormones—such as estrogen, progesterone, and testosterone—decline, our stress hormone, cortisol, tends to rise. All of this affects our skin texture and appearance. Don't fret: It's not a lost cause! There are ways to balance your hormones naturally, whatever your age.

ROOT CAUSE #4: NUTRITIONAL DEFICIENCIES

We need key nutrients to maintain healthy skin, and Sage-types tend to have nutritional deficiencies. For example, essential fatty acids help maintain skin cell hydration and function, and vitamin C helps build and maintain collagen. Deficiencies in these areas, among others, may stem from digestion and absorption issues, which will improve when you follow my recommendations.

While the gut microbiome may not have been the initial trigger for Sage-types, it certainly plays a role in our skin's microbiome and aging. Building up the gut and skin microbiomes can help us age gracefully.

WHAT TYPE ARE YOU?

As you read about these five skin types, you may relate to one or more. Many of my patients do. For example, my patient Sally is both an Amber and an Olivia. She struggled with acne as a teen, melasma during pregnancy, and then, at thirty-eight, started breaking out again. Another patient, Susan, is an Emmett and a Sage who has coped with eczema and dry skin challenges throughout her life. Now in her fifties, she's noticing sagging skin and excess wrinkles.

I relate to all of these skin types. At some point in my life, I have been an Amber, an Olivia, a Heath, an Emmett, and a Sage. Because of my Scottish-Irish genes, I have an Amber-like tendency to develop freckles. While some people may find freckles cute, they're a sign of skin damage, so it's important to address them. I'm not as much of an Olivia-type, but I've certainly had my fair share of acne breakouts, especially in my teens and twenties. I've identified with Heath, as I flushed and blushed easily as a child and then had a tendency to develop rosacea as an adult. Emmett was my identity for most of my childhood. I was hyperreactive, sensitive, and allergic, and I constantly experienced itchy rashes. Now in my forties, I know how challenging it feels to be like Sage and see more wrinkles staring back at me in the mirror.

The good news is that I know how to address these skin types. I've helped myself and thousands of patients unveil their triggers and optimize their health for glowing skin and vibrant health. Have you identified your skin type and root causes? If you need help, take my *Skin Quiz* at TheSkinQuiz.com.

CHAPTER 2

Conquering Skinflammation and Other Root Causes

In chapter 1, we covered the six root causes of skin problems and The Spa Dr.'s five skin types to help identify your weak spots. Now that we've identified the underlying triggers behind your skin issues, let's address them and begin your journey to achieving clear, glowing skin.

ADDRESSING YOUR ROOT CAUSES

In this chapter, I cover both external (environmental) and internal (biological) approaches. Conventional skin care treatments usually start and stop with external treatment. But traditionally trained estheticians and dermatologists are missing the most important step: what's happening *inside* the body. These internal approaches to addressing the problems are directly related to the six root causes that can lead to imperfect skin covered in chapter 1. To review, they are:

1. Inflammation

2. Microbiome disturbance

3. Oxidative damage

4. Blood sugar issues

5. Nutritional deficiencies

6. Hormonal imbalances

Now, let's address each one head on.

ADDRESSING ROOT CAUSE #1: INFLAMMATION

Addressing inflammation is one of the most crucial things you can do for your skin. When we reduce inflammation internally, skinflammation subsides and our skin clears. Inflammation also occurs externally, so we'll take a two-part approach to managing inflammation: inner and outer soothing.

Inner soothing addresses root causes that trigger inflammation internally. A key to this is avoiding foods that can cause inflammation, as well as choosing anti-inflammatory foods that can help calm inflammation and restore your body to its natural state. This also means balancing your immune response so your body isn't continuously preparing to fight.

When it comes to foods that inflame, some of the biggest triggers are food intolerances and allergies. Often when people think

> *"Addressing inflammation is one of the most crucial things you can do for your skin."*

of allergies, anaphylactic reactions such as hives, swollen lips, and difficulty breathing come to mind. Allergies occur when our bodies' immune systems see a substance as harmful and overreact to it, which creates a cascade of internal responses that sometimes lead to a life-threatening reaction. This response triggers immunoglobulins called IgEs, but there are also food sensitivities, whereby the body creates an immune response similar to an allergy, with different immunoglobulins involved. This reaction sets off an inflammatory response in the body. While the symptoms may not be as immediate or life-threatening, they are ongoing and can be debilitating in a different way. So when you eat a reactive food, it's like being exposed to a toxin—your body goes into attack mode and triggers a cascade of immune system reactions that next lead to inflammatory symptoms, which can appear on your skin.

FOOD SENSITIVITIES

Some of the most common skin reactions linked to food sensitivity include itching, flushing, red spots or bumps, acne, changes in perspiration odor, and worsening of skin conditions, such as psoriasis, eczema, infections, or vitiligo. Food sensitivities can also create a number of other symptoms. In chapter 3 I will cover the most common reactive foods and how to replace them with skin-nourishing, anti-inflammatory foods during my two-week program.

For Emmett-types (see pages 27–28), food allergies and sensitivities are particularly important to address, and one primary way is to avoid reactive foods.

THE GUT CONNECTION

Another important aspect when addressing inflammation is gut healing. As you learned in chapter 1, a major source of inflammation starts in the gut with "leaky gut syndrome," or hyperpermeability of the digestive tract lining, which kicks our immune system into overdrive. Avoiding reactive foods, addressing the gut microbiome, and getting proper nourishment, as well as other aspects of my two-week program, will enhance your digestive system and help repair a leaky gut.

Because diet is key in healing, I cover specific anti-inflammatory foods in more detail in later chapters. Examples of such foods include wild-caught fish, colorful fruits and vegetables, olives, and walnuts. Some of my favorite anti-inflammatory herbs and spices include turmeric, ginger, and rosemary. You'll learn how to incorporate these and other anti-inflammatory and natural flavor enhancers into your diet using my recipes (see chapters 7 and 8).

THE ENVIRONMENT

Contact with environmental toxins increases inflammation, so we need to reduce our exposure and boost our body's detoxification pathways to help clear the body. I will cover this further in the discussion of oxidative damage (see page 35) and the specifics in chapters 4 and 5.

If you're an Olivia, Heath, or Emmett skin type (see pages 25–28), you may need additional anti-inflammatory support from supplements. If your skin is inflamed, your insides probably are too. So squelch that internal inflammation with probiotics, omega-3s (EPA, or eicosapentaenoic acid), and other anti-inflammatory supplements, such as curcumin, bromelain, and boswellia.

CALMING THE SKIN

Because most chronic skin conditions are triggered by inflammation, it's imperative to do everything possible to calm the skin. *Externally* we can do that using ingredients found right in your kitchen, as well as with those found in high-quality, natural skin care products such as The Spa Dr. system.

However, many products we apply to our skin can actually exacerbate inflammation. Toxic skin care ingredients are pro-inflammatory, so refer to chapter 5 (see pages 77–79) for a full list of ingredients to eliminate from your skin care regimen and what to replace them with.

Two of my favorite natural ingredients are aloe and arnica. Aloe vera (*aloe barbadensis*) can effectively penetrate and transport healthy substances through the skin. Aloe is rich in mucopolysaccharides (naturally occurring sugars that keep skin moist and plump), minerals, amino acids, and enzymes. Aloe is renowned for its soothing, anti-inflammatory, and healing properties, making it suitable for remedying everything from cuts, scrapes, and sunburn to acne, dermatitis, and sensitive, irritated skin.

Arnica (*Arnica montana*) flower extract has powerful anti-inflammatory and anti-bacterial properties that can help alleviate pain and swelling and improve wound healing. If applied immediately after a trauma, it can prevent bruise formation by healing damaged capillaries. Skin-wise, arnica reduces the appearance of dark under-eye circles and dry, flaky, sensitive, blotchy skin.

These are two examples of natural actives that can reduce inflammation externally. There are many more to come!

ADDRESSING ROOT CAUSE #2: MICROBIOME DISTURBANCE

Because our skin microbiome is an extension of our gut microbiome, maintaining its balance is crucial. Even if you don't have digestive symptoms, there's still a good chance you have gut microbiome issues. And if you have chronic skin problems, such as acne or eczema, those conditions signal a skin microbiome imbalance.

If your skin is similar to that of Olivia, Heath, or Emmett (see pages 25–28), skin microbiome balance is particularly important for you. If you're an Amber (see pages 23–25) or a Sage (see pages 28–30), pay close attention too, because your skin microbiome affects your skin's youthfulness and overall appearance.

PROBIOTICS AND PREBIOTICS

Although "germs" often get a bad rap, some microorganisms are actually good for us. Those microorganisms—the *beneficial* bacteria—can be found in certain foods and can promote overall health, including your skin's quality. You can find these probiotic nutrients in fermented foods, such as kimchi, sauerkraut, pickled produce, yogurt, and kefir. *Prebiotic* foods—those that promote the growth of good bacteria in your gut—include dandelion greens, garlic, onions, leeks, and chicory. In chapters 4 and 8 I show you how to add these and other nourishing foods to your plate.

For some people, eating probiotic- and prebiotic-rich foods is not enough because their gut microbiome has already been compromised. If you have digestive symptoms (nausea, bloating, gassiness, heartburn, constipation, diarrhea), have more-intense chronic skin issues, or have taken a heavy course, or multiple courses, of antibiotics or oral steroids, it is likely you need additional support. Often, taking a high-quality probiotic supplement will help you get back on track. If your issues continue, I highly recommend seeing a licensed naturopathic physician or functional medicine doctor who can do specialized testing.

For example, one test I often run is the comprehensive digestive stool analysis test, which can offer insight into an individual's imbalances, overgrowth, or deficiencies of various bacteria, as well as yeasts, parasites, and other bugs that dwell in our intestines. This information can help tailor treatment. If you have parasites or an overgrowth of candida, yeast, or bacteria, your practitioner will give you specific herbal or nutritional supplements, maybe even prescription medications, to address these issues. Until that's done, restoring balance to the gut microbiome will be challenging.

For most people, eating probiotic- and prebiotic-rich foods and cutting excess carbohydrates and sugars from your diet is sufficient to restore microbiome balance and set the stage for beautiful, clear skin. Some of you will have to work a bit harder, but everything I explain in the two-week program will help.

A BALANCED SKIN MICROBIOME

On the outside, our skin microbiome is also important (and often overlooked). The exterior of human skin has a natural pH level of about 4 to 4.5. A pH below 7 is considered acidic; a pH above 7 is considered alkaline. Skin's mild acidity helps keep it hydrated and healthy. However, what you put on your skin greatly affects its pH and can easily throw things off balance.

For many years there was a misbelief that balanced pH for skin was a neutral level of 6 to 7, but research now suggests that number should actually be under 5. A mildly acidic environment keeps skin's microbiome in balance; a more alkaline pH (around 8 to 9) kills or disrupts that balance. Many common skin care products are alkaline and can increase skin's pH.

Even water is too alkaline for skin. After water touches your skin, I suggest rebalancing the pH to a mildly acidic level using high-quality skin care products. Cleansers, toners, serums, and moisturizers with a pH of 5.5 and higher can dry out your skin and make it more prone to infections, outbreaks, and premature aging.

A skin care product's formula helps determine its pH, and while it might seem as though you'd have to add synthetic ingredients to make it more acidic, there are many natural ingredients that reduce the pH to the mildly acidic range. Citric acid, for example, achieves this and is naturally occurring in citrus fruits. Not all natural skin care products are made with mild acidity in mind, so it is important to look closely at the label and ask questions. Sometimes the pH is listed; if it's not, contact the manufacturer to find out. The Spa Dr. skin care line embraces this science.

In addition, there are oils that help promote mild acidity and have other balancing effects for skin. Argan kernel oil is extracted from the kernels of the Moroccan argan tree (*Argania spinosa*). It can restore resilience to the acid mantle and impart luminosity, softness, and moisture to skin, as well as protect against dryness. Argan oil is chock-full of vitamin E, fatty acids (vitamin F), carotenoids such as beta-carotene, and phytosterols. Argan oil is a noncomedogenic (nonclogging), anti-inflammatory, and regenerative agent—so it's good for oily and acne-prone skin types.

OUR COMPLETE MICROBIOME

Our body does an amazing job controlling internal pH, especially when given the right foods and nutrients. Eating a nourishing, plant-focused diet will help your body remain pH balanced internally. But, as you can see, both the gut and the skin microbiomes play a big role in skin health. When both are properly balanced, we see the difference in clear, youthful-looking skin. If you've struggled with skin issues for years, especially if you've taken or used topical or oral antibiotics and steroids or stripped your skin with invasive procedures, this is likely one primary cause you'll address. My two-week program is designed for people like you!

ADDRESSING ROOT CAUSE #3:
OXIDATIVE DAMAGE

You're aware of the damage that sun exposure and tobacco smoke can have on your complexion, but we are exposed to a number of other toxins on a daily basis *internally* that harm our organs, including the skin. Exposure to chemical toxins in your air, water, and food can trigger oxidative damage, as well as other root causes, including inflammation, microbiome disturbance, nutritional deficiencies, and hormone imbalances.

> *"Whatever your skin type, toxin exposure is a primary trigger, and avoiding toxins is essential for clear, glowing skin."*

Whatever your skin type, toxin exposure is a primary trigger, and avoiding toxins is essential for clear, glowing skin.

Unfortunately, the number of chemicals and toxins in our environment is increasing at an alarming rate, and our bodies soak them up like sponges. When it rains, air pollutants, pesticides, and other chemicals are washed into our water supply. The crops we eat absorb this water, which exposes us further. The animals we eat also live off the contaminated water, plants, and feed, so chemicals concentrate in their bodies. When we eat this meat and fish, we further come in contact with toxins. We have become human storage tanks for chemicals, and we now know it's not a matter of *if* but *how* these toxins affect us.

One toxin of particular concern is endocrine-disrupting chemicals (EDCs). EDCs include substances in our environment, water, food, and personal care products that interfere with the production, transport, breakdown, binding, and elimination of hormones. Exposure to EDCs ultimately affects the hormonal system and the body's homeostasis and, thus, the skin.

The most effective way you can avoid the harmful effects of these chemicals is to eliminate exposure entirely. This means choosing clean water, food, personal care products, and other items in our immediate environment. My two-week program addresses this.

FOCUS ON SKIN CARE

In the United States, skin care products are not well regulated or screened for true safety. While the European Union (EU) has banned hundreds of ingredients in personal care products, the U.S. Food and Drug Administration (FDA) has banned only eleven ingredients.

Research shows that many chemical ingredients are hormone disruptors and that some may even be carcinogenic. We're exposed to these chemicals when we inhale them from sprays and powders, ingest them from the lips, and absorb them through our skin. Statistics suggest women use an average of twelve personal care products daily, while men use an average of six. Based on the average number of ingredients in a personal care product, we're exposed to an average of 126 different ingredients daily. Our skin is highly sensitive to the inflammatory effects of these chemicals, and that can have a huge effect on our appearance.

The preservatives, fragrances, and other common ingredients in personal care products are known to contain a number of EDCs. Because research links EDCs with certain conditions, such as thyroid problems, infertility, early puberty, obesity, diabetes, and certain types of cancer (such as prostate and breast), avoid these ingredients.

Our hormones change as we age, and this contributes to accelerated fine lines and wrinkles in our thirties, forties, and beyond. So why would we throw our hormones even further out of balance with exposure to EDCs? Some of the most concerning EDCs are phthalates in fragrance, formaldehyde-releasers, oxybenzone in sunscreen, and parabens, which are used as preservatives.

In addition to toxic chemicals, many products contain genetically modified or irradiated ingredients and common allergens, such as gluten. I give you a full list of ingredients to avoid and discuss personal care products further in chapter 3. In the meantime, keep in mind that what you put on your body can penetrate your skin and end up in your bloodstream; it's time to take a closer look at ingredient labels.

DETOXIFYING OUR BODIES

While toxins are unavoidable, there is a way to detoxify our systems and preserve our skin health. Not only are the body's detoxification pathways essential for dumping toxins—they're also important for keeping our hormones balanced. Our liver and kidneys are amazing tools for removing toxins, but when overexposure to toxins occurs and that contact is coupled with underlying genetic factors and a possible combination of organ impairment, our systems may become overloaded and can malfunction. Even with our body's great cleansing abilities, we sometimes need to offer it extra support to ensure optimal functioning. The first step is reducing exposure to toxins. Next you will ensure your body is balanced and decrease inflammation for proper organ function. Then you'll rev up your detoxification pathways.

On a daily basis, the best way to do that is by consuming cleansing foods and nutrients. My favorite cleansing foods are cruciferous vegetables (turnips, cabbage, kale, brussels sprouts, cauliflower, collards, mustard greens, radishes, and rutabaga), onions, garlic, and fermented foods. The glucosinolates in cruciferous vegetables—in particular indole-3-carbinol, sulforaphane, diindolylmethane (DIM), and

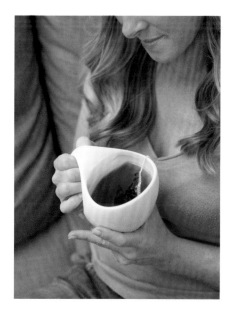

particular, is one of the primary biological processes for removing toxins from the skin. We want our skin to be detoxed and exfoliated regularly to help ease this elimination route.

Desquamation, shedding the skin's outer layer, normally occurs every fourteen days, but some of us need extra support to ensure that turnover happens.

If your skin is chronically dry, flaky, or bumpy—or really anything less than clear and glowing—you may need extra exfoliation support. This actually applies to most skin types, because most of us don't have soft, smooth, blemish-free skin. In chapter 3 we'll discuss how to achieve a clean slate by cleaning the skin.

For now I'll share two examples of natural ingredients that can help detox your skin.

isothiocyanate—enhance antioxidant properties and improve liver detoxification. Indole-3-carbinole increases the liver's ability to metabolize estrogen by almost 50 percent. Garlic and onions contain sulfur compounds, such as allicin, that support detoxification pathways. You can also drink herbal teas (dandelion, chicory, and milk thistle) to support kidney and liver function.

Regardless of your skin type, if you regularly experience digestive issues, headaches, fatigue, and irritability, then cleansing is particularly important. You may need to bump up the detox support with supplements, such as milk thistle, NAC (N-acetyl cysteine from the amino acid L-cysteine), and vitamin C. The two-week program explains more about how to personalize your program.

When you think about the body's main detoxifying organs, the skin probably doesn't come to mind. But skin actually plays an important role in this process. Sweating, in

1. Pineapple (*Ananas sativus*) fruit extract provides pineapple's bioactive properties. Pineapple is a natural source of bromelain, a proteolytic enzyme that digests proteins. Bromelain hydrolyzes proteins and digests only the dead cells on the skin's surface, leaving the living cells beneath intact and making this ingredient suitable for even the most sensitive skin types. Ultimately, pineapple extract offers an anti-inflammatory effect.

2. Green algae (*Chlorella vulgaris*) extract is a freshwater algae. It's used for its natural chelating properties (the ability to bind to and remove heavy metals) and high protein content. Chlorella contains nineteen to twenty-two essential and nonessential amino acids and a respectable amount of vitamins. When used topically, its beneficial properties help purify and energize skin.

TIPS FOR HEALTHY ELIMINATION

If your exit route for eliminating waste is closed (i.e., you are constipated), then your body is not able to get rid of these elements—toxins included. When this occurs, you are more likely to feel sluggish, tired, and irritable, and you may develop skin issues. You need to ensure you're not constipated before starting the two-week program. Here are some tips to unblock your exit route.

1. Drink more filtered water. Six to eight glasses (8 ounces, or 235 ml each) of filtered water daily will work well for most people, but some people need closer to ten glasses.

2. Increase your fiber intake. Fiber improves digestion, blood sugar balance, nutrient absorption, and intestinal microflora balance. It decreases intestinal transit time (it moves things along faster in our bowels), and increases the weight and size of stools, which is healthier for the colon. Health experts recommend 25 to 30 grams of fiber per day, but most people get only about 10 grams or less. To ensure you're consuming at least 25 grams per day, eat:

- 6 or more servings of vegetables
- 1 to 2 servings of legumes
- 1 to 2 servings of fruit
- 1 serving of whole grains
- You may also consider a supplement, such as ground chia, flax, or psyllium.

3. Eat more fermented veggies, and take a probiotic supplement.

4. If the first three steps don't help, **take 400 mg of magnesium citrate.**

5. If that doesn't work, **take 3,000 to 6,000 mg of vitamin C.**

6. If nothing works, **take an herbal laxative, and consider seeing your health care provider.** It's not normal to be constipated to any degree—if you do not have at least one bowel movement a day, regularly, something is wrong.

These are just two examples of natural actives that cleanse your skin; there are many more. In addition to these ingredients, you can gently exfoliate your skin with my DIY facials (see pages 176–190).

ADDRESSING ROOT CAUSE #4: BLOOD SUGAR ISSUES

Keeping your blood sugar in check is essential for skin health. As mentioned earlier, during glycation, sugar in the bloodstream can attach to proteins to form AGEs (see page 21), and AGEs accelerate skin aging. If you are a Sage-type (see pages 25–26), this is particularly important for you.

To review what we've learned, elevated blood sugar increases insulin and androgen activity and causes acne. This is a big trigger for Olivia-types (see pages 25–26), but blood sugar affects us all. Sugar is an acidic, pro-inflammatory food—neither of which is good for our skin or overall health.

To maintain healthy blood sugar levels, cut back on sugars or anything that turns to sugar in the body. "Sugar" comes in many forms, from corn syrup, cane or beet sugar, and fructose to honey, agave syrup, and maple syrup (and more!). All elevate blood sugar and lead to the problems previously discussed. I know what you're thinking . . . how can I give up sweets? Don't worry; I give you super-tasty healthier alternatives that will satisfy your sweet tooth.

When it comes to achieving glowing skin, reducing sugar consumption goes hand in hand with eating balanced meals throughout the day. I'll explain how to "balance your plate" so you will know what ratio of macronutrients—protein, fats, and carbohydrates—each meal and snack should have. The great news is, when you shift your plate,

you'll automatically increase your fiber intake, which is critical for keeping blood sugar balanced.

For most people, dietary changes are all that are needed to balance blood sugar. To determine whether you need extra support, I recommend having blood work done by your health care provider. I, along with most doctors, recommend getting routine blood work at least every two years, more frequently if you have any serious or chronic illness, or if your blood work reveals anything suboptimal. During routine blood work, doctors usually check blood glucose, but it's always good to request this. If you are an Olivia- or Sage-type (see pages 25–26 or 28–30) and haven't had your blood sugar checked in more than a year, I highly recommend scheduling an appointment.

Ask your doctor to order a fasting blood glucose test. If you have a history of elevated blood sugar or your doctor is willing to let you take the test, include HbgA1C and insulin, as well. Fasting blood glucose indicates your blood sugar level the moment your blood is drawn, while HgbA1C indicates where your blood sugar has been over an extended period of time. The hormone insulin helps transport the blood sugar. Your insulin level reading can provide important information about how your body is regulating your blood sugar levels.

When you have blood drawn, request a copy of your blood work. Your practitioner may tell you all is "normal" (which is usually considered below 100), but I want your levels to be optimal, which means under 85. If your levels are over 85, or your HgbA1C or insulin is out of normal range, you'll want extra support for blood sugar balance.

You can optimize your blood sugar with certain nutrients, such as chromium, fiber, and alpha lipoic acid, as well as herbs, such as gymnema and bitter melon. However, if you have been diagnosed with diabetes or your doctor says your blood levels are abnormal, it's important to work with a licensed health care provider to get those in check. High or low blood sugar can have serious short-term and long-term health implications. If that's the case for you, your doctor should be closely monitoring those levels.

ADDRESSING ROOT CAUSE #5: NUTRITIONAL DEFICIENCIES

A nutrient-rich diet helps ensure a healthy glow and promotes graceful aging.

Nutritional deficiencies often are the result of poor dietary and lifestyle habits, absorption issues, or a lack of nutrients in our diet. When it comes to skin, in addition to water and protein consumption, specific nutrients not only address deficiencies but also enhance skin quality. There are a number of micronutrients that play a role in our skin health, and I've identified eight that are the most important nutrients for skin. These are:

1. Essential fatty acids (EFAs)

2. Vitamin D

3. Vitamin C

4. Zinc

5. Vitamin E

6. Vitamin A

7. B vitamins

8. Probiotics

ESSENTIAL FATTY ACIDS

Essential fatty acids (EFAs) cannot be synthesized within the body, so they must be obtained through diet. There are two main types of essential fatty acids: omega-3s and omega-6s. They're unsaturated fats found in plants and fatty fishes.

For healthy bodies and skin, omega-3 and omega-6 fatty acids must be consumed in the right ratio. While *some* omega-6 fatty acid consumption is good, most people consume too much omega-6-rich food (usually in the form of vegetable oils) in relationship to omega-3s. The ratio of omega-6 to omega-3 consumption is commonly 10:1 to 20:1, when it should be closer to 1:1 or 2:1.

The best source of omega-3s is fish, such as wild Alaskan salmon. But it can be found in other forms too, which is good news if you don't like fish. Other sources include grass-fed beef, flaxseed, walnuts, and eggs from free-range chickens. You can also get a dose of omega-3s by taking a high-quality supplement. While I'm not opposed to a vegetarian diet, flaxseed and walnuts have to be converted into omega-3s in the body, so fish provides a more direct source.

Omega-3s are scientifically shown to promote heart health and even reduce depressive symptoms. They also have an imperative function when it comes to skin health: reducing inflammation. This specific nutrient can help remedy inflammatory skin issues, such as atopic dermatitis, psoriasis, and acne, and in turn provide glowing results.

Research also suggests that fish oil reduces levels of leukotriene B4, a substance linked to eczema. Therapeutic dosage recommendations for adults range from 200 mg EPA to 2 to 4 grams total omega-3s.

VITAMIN D

Sun exposure is a great way to get your fix of vitamin D—a nutrient in which most Americans are deficient. Knowing how much sun exposure you need for the right amount of vitamin D depends on a number of variables—from where you live to how much pigmentation your skin has. However, research shows that simply standing in the sun for up to thirty minutes twice a week with arms and legs exposed, during late morning to late afternoon, can often provide the recommended vitamin D intake.

Because being in the sun releases endorphins and makes us feel good—and because the tanned look is perceived as fashionable—many of us get too much sun and harm our skin in the process. Excess UV ray exposure causes oxidative damage, affecting DNA and leaving the body at a heightened risk of melanoma and other types of skin cancer, not to mention accelerating aging.

Although called a vitamin, vitamin D is technically a hormone because our bodies produce it in response to sunlight exposure on skin. We get vitamin D from exposure to sunlight (vitamin D_3), but also from our diet (vitamins D_3 and D_2) and supplements (vitamins D_3 and D_2)—*but I always recommend D_3*. Vitamin D helps manage skin conditions such as atopic dermatitis, psoriasis, vitiligo, acne, and rosacea, and it can protect skin from the sun's UV damage.

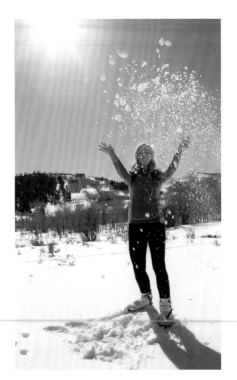

The best sources of vitamin D are:

▸ Cod liver oil: 1 teaspoon = 400 to 1,000 international units (IU) of vitamin D_3

▸ Egg yolk: 20 IU of vitamin D_3 or D_2

▸ Shiitake mushrooms (sun-dried): 3.5 ounces (100 g) = 1,600 IU of vitamin D_2

▸ Sunlight exposure: 5 to 30 minutes' exposure to arms and legs twice per week (without sunscreen) = vitamin D_3 (amount varies depending upon location, season, duration, and pigmentation); *I recommend wearing a hat, sunglasses, and a mineral-based sunblock on your face any time you're in the sun.*

▸ Supplements: vitamin D_3 (amount varies depending on supplement)

▸ Wild, fresh salmon: 3.5 ounces (100 g) = 600 to 1,000 IU of vitamin D_3

WHAT FACTORS DECREASE OUR VITAMIN D LEVELS?

If you're worried about a vitamin D deficiency, your doctor can order 25-hydroxy vitamin D as part of your blood work. Vitamin D from the skin and diet is metabolized in the liver to 25-hydroxy vitamin D. This is the best marker for vitamin D status, as it best reflects vitamin D stores and indicates how much the skin is making and how much your body is consuming.

- Aging (Vitamin D production reduces as we age.)

- Breastfeeding

- Geographic location (Above 35 degrees north latitude, little to no vitamin D can be produced from November to February.)

- Health conditions that create malabsorption and lead to certain conditions, such as celiac disease and Crohn's disease; other health conditions, such as hyperthyroidism

- Liver dysfunction and kidney disease

- Living in a city with high smog levels (Visit www.airnow.gov to learn about the air quality of your hometown.)

- Medications, such as those that reduce cholesterol absorption

- Obesity

- Season (Little to no vitamin D is made in winter months.)

- Skin pigmentation (Darker skin reduces production of vitamin D by up to 99 percent.)

- Sunscreen use and protective clothing (SPF 15 reduces vitamin D synthesis by 99 percent.)

VITAMIN C

You've probably scanned the skin care aisle at your local drugstore and seen vitamin C splashed across labels, hailing antiaging and skin-brightening effects. Vitamin C can be found in supplement form, as well as in a number of fruits and vegetables—including oranges, cantaloupe, watercress, bell peppers, strawberries, and broccoli. Getting your vitamin C fix is crucial because it is vital for collagen synthesis, and some research shows it can even help reverse UV damage to skin. While vitamin C isn't a sunscreen (it doesn't absorb the sun's UVA or UVB rays), its antioxidant feature helps combat the effects of free radicals.

Vitamin C is a natural component in the skin's dermis and epidermis (above the dermis) layers, but as you age—you guessed it—production of the antioxidant begins to lag. Excess sun exposure and smoking can cause vitamin C levels to fall in the epidermis, in particular. Because vitamin C aids in building collagen, it can help prevent the formation of wrinkles. We also know vitamin C deficiency causes easy bruising, poor wound healing, and loss of skin tone and elasticity. If you're a Sage-type (see pages 28–30), in particular, be sure to get vitamin C in your diet, and consider a supplement for extra support. Many recipes in this book are rich in vitamin C.

ZINC

Zinc has been used as a nutrient in skin therapy for centuries, and it's known for its wound healing and anti-inflammatory properties. Zinc is prevalent in the epidermis, and zinc deficiencies have been shown to lead to a number of skin problems, such as dermatitis and leg ulcers.

Superficially, zinc oxide is often a key ingredient in sunblocks and soothing agents. It is used topically to treat a number of skin conditions, including dandruff, dermatitis, warts, fungal skin infections, acne, rosacea, and melasma. Research shows that oral zinc is also an essential micronutrient for skin growth and repair, as well as for helping a host of other skin problems. Our need for zinc appears to increase as we age. In your diet you can get zinc from eggs, meat, and seafood. If you're vegan, you may be deficient in this skin-essential nutrient.

VITAMIN E

Vitamin E is one of the best-known nutrients thought to be essential for a healthy complexion. Vitamin E oil for skin, applied externally, boasts benefits including the ability to reduce wrinkles, stretch marks, fine lines, and brown spots. It also possesses wound-healing properties, and some people use it to nourish dry or cracked cuticles.

Adding vitamin E to your diet can lead to equally impressive results. Because vitamin E is an antioxidant, it can help fight premature aging by protecting cells from free radical damage—which, as you've already learned, results from air pollution, smoking, and excess sun exposure. Foods rich in vitamin E include olive oil, sunflower seeds, almonds, hazelnuts, leafy greens such as turnip greens, and avocados.

VITAMIN A

Vitamin A helps prevent premature wrinkles and bumpy skin. It is found in egg yolks and liver, dark leafy greens, and, in the carotenoid form, in dark orange or green veggies and fruits, such as carrots and sweet potatoes. If you eat liver, make sure you get it from a clean source, such as organic free-range chicken.

Like vitamin E, vitamin A is a fat-soluble vitamin with antiaging and healing properties for skin. Acne and dry or scaly skin are all potential signs of vitamin A deficiency, but supplements can help repair these symptoms. Also similar to vitamin E, known for its healing properties, vitamin A aids in tissue rebuilding, and can be the perfect remedy for wounds and scrapes.

Commercially, vitamin A has gotten attention because its active form, retinoids, can treat acne, psoriasis, eczema, and cold sores, as well as aging-related skin problems, such as wrinkles, fine lines, and dark spots. But while vitamin A protects from UV rays, retinoids can actually increase sun exposure damage. If you use one of these products, avoid applying too much before going out in the sun when exposure is at its peak.

Carotenoids, dark-colored pigments in produce, have been shown to reduce the risk of cancer and are processed as a form of vitamin A in the body. Beta-carotene, a carotenoid, is an antioxidant, so it protects skin from free radicals and signs of aging.

Beta-carotene is found in brightly colored yellow and orange fruits and vegetables, such as apricots, cantaloupe, carrots, sweet potatoes, and winter squash. Leafy greens, such as spinach and broccoli, also contain carotenoids. The richer the produce's color, the greater the beta-carotene it provides.

B VITAMINS

If you scan the vitamin aisle at your drugstore or health food store, you'll find various vitamin B options. While many of them can do the body good, there are a few you should focus on specifically to enhance your skin: biotin (vitamin B7), pantothenic acid (vitamin B5), and niacin (vitamin B3).

You'll often find biotin in multivitamins, B-complex, and skin support supplements because biotin is thought to play a crucial role in maintaining healthy skin, hair, and nails. The first signs of biotin deficiency usually appear on our skin (such as a red, scaly rash around the eyes, nose, and mouth). Like the other B vitamins, it's water soluble rather than fat soluble, so it doesn't accumulate in our tissues. Biotin helps the enzymes that break down fats and carbohydrates convert fuel into energy. Food sources of biotin include bananas, cauliflower, egg yolks, legumes, liver, mushrooms, Swiss chard, and watermelon.

Often found in moisturizers, vitamin B5 can help stabilize the skin's barrier, promote skin softness and elasticity, and reduce inflammation and redness. The nutrient also holds clout as a healer because vitamin B5 can soothe minor cuts and scrapes, rashes, bedsores, acne, eczema, and dermatitis. A 2002 study in the *Journal of Dermatological Treatment* noted that vitamin B5 enhanced the repair of the skin barrier while reducing inflammation. You can find vitamin B5 in organic meats, eggs, broccoli, fish, shellfish, chicken, mushrooms, avocado, legumes, and sweet potatoes.

If you have acne, niacin (vitamin B3) is one micronutrient you surely want, as it is known for its capability to banish this skin woe. Chicken, eggs, fish, meat, legumes, and seeds are all good sources of niacin. In the body, niacin is converted to niacinamide, the active form of the vitamin. Niacinamide is used topically and taken internally to help reduce wrinkles, pigmentation (melasma), rosacea, and sebum production (acne).

In general, if you take any B-vitamin supplement long term, it's best to take a well-rounded approach with a B-complex or a multiple B-vitamin supplement. All the B vitamins have their benefits, and most work well synergistically.

PROBIOTICS

We've already covered how enhancing digestion helps address most skin care issues. So it makes sense that probiotics are part of that. Probiotics are well known for their intestine-aiding abilities—they help maintain equilibrium in the body, including the "good" and "bad" bacteria in the gut microbiome. Anxiety, stress, and a diet low in fiber and high in processed foods can affect that balance and increase the chance of skinflammation, leading to myriad skin problems.

Consuming probiotics, considered "good" bacteria, has been shown to reverse those effects by restoring balance in the gut. This truth spans decades: A report by R. H. Siver published in 1961 indicated that among 300 acne patients given a probiotic, 80 percent saw their acne improve. Similarly, a study by Kim et al. published in 2010 in the journal *Nutrition* revealed that fifty-six people suffering from acne who consumed a lactobacillus-fermented drink for twelve weeks had less oily secretions and fewer acne lesions.

Adding probiotics to the diet can also alleviate rosacea. Science shows they may reduce symptoms such as redness, pimples, and dryness that result from the condition. Probiotics have also been used as a treatment for psoriasis, and consuming them has been linked to a reduced chance of developing eczema in studies of children whose families had a history of the disease.

Probiotics also can ultimately boost collagen production in skin, a powerful antiaging component that increases elasticity and can help reduce sun damage. Probiotics can be found in fermented drinks, yogurt with live active cultures, sauerkraut, kimchi, and miso soup.

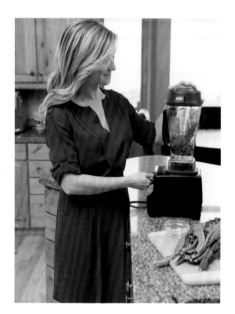

TOTAL NOURISHMENT

Balanced nutrients are crucial for healthy skin. Because no single vitamin, be it biotin or vitamin E, is found alone organically, it's always a good idea to mimic nature when we think of nutrients. This way we'll maintain that essential and intricate balance, and see the effects we desire. That's why I recommend getting the majority of your nutrients from food. And for many people I recommend adding a high-quality multivitamin/mineral supplement. If you suspect you have digestive/absorption issues or you have a nutrient-deficient diet, it's time to include a multivitamin as part of your daily regimen.

Let's not forget that nourishing our bodies occurs on the outside too. There's a lot of hype in skin care marketing, but many popular skin care products do not contain what they claim, and the nutrients they do include are often not the highest quality or supplied in optimal amounts.

There's more research now than ever before on naturally nourishing ingredients. We know certain ingredients, such as green tea extract, CoQ10, and vitamin C, have great skin benefits. Many skin care companies now use some natural ingredients, but if you look closely at the label (if you can find it!), you'll probably find many other synthetic ingredients there. In the end, these are not truly natural, so in addition to the natural ingredients, you're exposed to the same toxins discussed earlier.

It's also important to know where the raw materials come from and how much is actually in the product. Most skin care products contain such a small amount of the natural ingredients that they're not actually effective. Manufacturers may use a very weak version of isolated nutrients. This prevents the products from doing what research shows natural ingredients can do. Unfortunately, this is one reason we often hear conventional dermatologists dismiss the efficacy of natural skin care products.

We know kale and other greens are good for our health, but quality and quantity matter. If we're eating canned greens or only a pinch of fresh greens each day, we're not getting sufficient amounts of greens. Similarly, with skin care ingredients, if you do not obtain the right amounts and strengths of the potent natural actives, you miss out on their benefits.

Throughout this book, I talk about ingredients you can find in your kitchen and what to look for in natural skin care products. For now, I'll highlight a few potent natural actives that nourish your skin externally.

- **Pichia/resveratrol ferment extract** is made from grapes and fermented with the pichia yeast. This potent antioxidant delivers scientifically tested and proven

health and antiaging benefits. Clinical research has identified how free radicals contribute to cell destruction, and because cell damage is at the root of most aging disorders, protecting skin from free radical activity is a significant preventive measure for healthy skin.

- **Ubiquinone (CoQ10)** is a powerful natural active; found in all living cells, it is essential for cell metabolism. It has been studied extensively to establish its safety and beneficial properties, both when ingested and when applied topically. Ubiquinone is known for its powerful antioxidant properties, along with its role in cell energy. Clinical studies report its ability to reduce the depth of wrinkles and accelerate collagen production—thereby gaining it a reputation as an antiaging active. It's important to use an all-natural, high-purity form of ubiquinone produced by yeast fermentation (synthetic sources have been found to contain impurities), which is identical to what is naturally produced in the body, making it more readily bioavailable to the skin.

- **Sea buckthorn (_Hippophae rhamnoides_) fruit oil** is an effective rejuvenating agent that can help stimulate microcirculation and cell regeneration. This active also can help combat inflammation. Sea buckthorn seed oil is the only plant known to contain omega-3s, omega-6s, omega-9s—and the rare omega-7—all together. It also contains a vitamin C concentration ten times greater than an orange's. Just as EFAs and vitamin C are nourishing internally, they're also great when used externally on skin.

ADDRESSING ROOT CAUSE #6:
HORMONAL IMBALANCES

Hormones are important chemical messengers produced in organs, such as the ovaries, adrenal glands, and thyroid glands, and they play a big role in your overall health and your skin's health.

You can support hormonal balance by managing stress, eating a balanced and nutrient-rich diet, getting a good night's rest, and exercising regularly. Aid liver detoxification pathways to help ensure proper hormone metabolism by eating cruciferous vegetables, onions, and garlic. My two-week program supports and guides you through the foods and lifestyle changes that promote this.

There are four hormones that affect your skin in big ways:

1. Estrogen

2. Testosterone

3. Thyroid hormones

4. Cortisol

Let's examine each briefly to better understand its effects.

ESTROGEN

Estrogen levels decrease as we age, which creates significant changes in the skin, including dry, wrinkle-prone, less elastic, more fragile, and even paler skin. The biggest culprit of sagging skin and loss of hydration (particularly among women over age forty) is declining estrogen levels. With a sudden drop in estrogen, skin appears thin, sallow, and saggy. Most notably, fine lines will turn into deep creases. The areas around the eyes and lips droop slightly and lose firmness. Your

> *"You can support hormonal balance by managing stress, eating a balanced and nutrient-rich diet, getting a good night's rest, and exercising regularly."*

skin will also not look as vibrant because less blood flow enters the skin.

If you're a Sage-type (see pages 28–30) or over forty and have any of the following symptoms, you may need additional estrogen support: bone loss, hot flashes, insomnia, mood changes, night sweats, or vaginal dryness.

Phytoestrogens (plant estrogens) can be found naturally in certain foods, such as flaxseed, and have been shown to have beneficial hormonal effects. Although flaxseed is known as a natural estrogen mimicker, eating flaxseed actually aids estrogen metabolism. This breakdown and removal of estrogens helps avoid excess levels.

Herbs such as maca, black cohosh, and hops also have been shown to help women low in estrogen. Some women also benefit from bio-identical hormone therapy (BHT). BHT requires the support of a well-trained hormone specialist.

High estrogen levels, on the other hand, come with their own problems. Women who are pregnant or on birth control pills generally have higher estrogen levels and are more prone to hyperpigmentation (also known as melasma). If you're an Amber-type (see pages 23–25) and taking hormones or experiencing melasma, be sure to balance your hormones, especially estrogen.

If your estrogen levels are too high, consider eating seaweed and cruciferous veggies (broccoli and kale), seasoning foods with turmeric, and taking supplements such as DIM (diindolylmethane, which comes from cruciferous vegetables); these can help with estrogen metabolism.

If you think your estrogen levels may be out of balance, talk with a qualified health care provider about testing your hormone levels and getting individualized support.

TESTOSTERONE

Testosterone stimulates the sebum-producing glands, which are important for protecting skin with natural oils, but in excess this hormone can lead to acne breakouts. Whether you're a man or a woman, hormones such as estrogen, progesterone, and testosterone help the body maintain a delicate balance. Sometimes hormone fluctuations during or around age-based shifts such as puberty and menopause lead to an increase in testosterone or challenges with hormone metabolism, which can lead to acne. If you are an Olivia-type (see pages 25–26) or your skin is excessively oily or prone to acne, you might be dealing with a testosterone imbalance.

One way to help testosterone balance and metabolism, and curb excess sebum production, is to avoid dairy products—even organic or raw. Dairy products are made from the milk of pregnant (and recently pregnant) cows, which contains hormones that can throw our own hormones out of balance.

I also recommend consuming omega-3s (in fish and supplements) and zinc, which you can consume via a supplement or get from green beans, sesame seeds, and pumpkin seeds. If you still have trouble with excess sebum and breakouts, supplementing with saw palmetto may aid testosterone metabolism, but it's important to check with your health care provider before overloading on supplements.

Supplementing with testosterone and DHEA (a hormone that converts, in part, to testosterone) increases the size and secretion of sebaceous glands. If your doctor has prescribed these for you and you have acne, check to ensure you're on the correct treatment regimen.

THYROID HORMONES

Thyroid hormones also influence your skin's appearance. Overactive thyroid can cause a warm, smooth, sweaty, and flushed skin. Underactive thyroid can lead to dry, coarse skin and a reduced ability to sweat.

If you experience any of these skin problems and have weight issues, digestion issues (constipation or diarrhea), or energy issues (fatigue or feeling overly stimulated), talk with your doctor about thyroid testing. If your thyroid is low or high, or you have antibodies, you'll want your treatment tailored accordingly.

The tests to ask for are TSH (thyroid stimulating hormone), Free T3, Free T4, and, if you can, thyroid antibodies and reverse T3.

To keep skin hydrated with a healthy oil barrier, consume essential fatty acids, such as omega-3s. A diet short of these body-nourishing fats can leave your skin dry, itchy, and prone to acne.

CORTISOL

When you're stressed, cortisol is released from your adrenal glands. A surge in cortisol increases sebum production, which triggers acne. It also amps up inflammatory pathways, which can exacerbate almost any skin issue. Chronically high levels of cortisol can also lead to sugar cravings, and eating sugar increases skinflammation and breakouts.

Stress comes in many forms, and it's not all bad. Our bodies are well equipped to handle acute stress, and this physical response helps us react quickly to dangerous situations—but balance is key. Problems occur when the body is exposed to repeated or continuous stress. At that point, the body has a hard time maintaining homeostasis and will continue to trigger physical reactions—eventually overwhelming our systems.

Chronic stress can worsen issues such as acne, eczema, rosacea, and vitiligo. Relaxation techniques such as breath work, moderate exercise, and meditation can effectively manage stress, especially when you make them a daily practice. In my two-week program, we'll talk about specific, powerful stress-busting techniques.

If you're overly stressed and often feel wired or tired, you may have imbalances in cortisol, or adrenal fatigue. You may notice you've gained extra weight around your midsection or have sugar cravings or insomnia. When that happens, you'll need extra support for your adrenals to balance your cortisol levels. Adaptogenic herbs such as rhodiola, ashwagandha, astragalus, and ginseng can help. You may want to talk with your health care provider about salivary cortisol testing. Even if you have imbalances in cortisol, the recommendations in this book will help support your adrenal function.

Also, using products containing adaptogenic herbs can help. For example, Ginseng (*Eleutherococcus senticosus*) root extract

"To keep skin hydrated with a healthy oil barrier, consume essential fatty acids, such as omega-3s."

can be topically applied to skin to create balance. Ginseng is a powerful adaptogen that increases the overall resistance to all types of stress and helps rejuvenate and invigorate tired-looking skin.

Many other hormones play a role in your skin health, but these are the major contributors for most skin types.

A LOOK AHEAD

When you address your specific root causes, you're on your way to clear, glowing skin. The next three chapters cover how to create a clean plate for optimal nourishment (chapter 3), a clean slate with external skin care (chapter 4), and a clean body for healthy detoxification pathways and a clean mind (chapter 5) for accelerated healing on another level. Then I'll help you bring it all together in my two-week program.

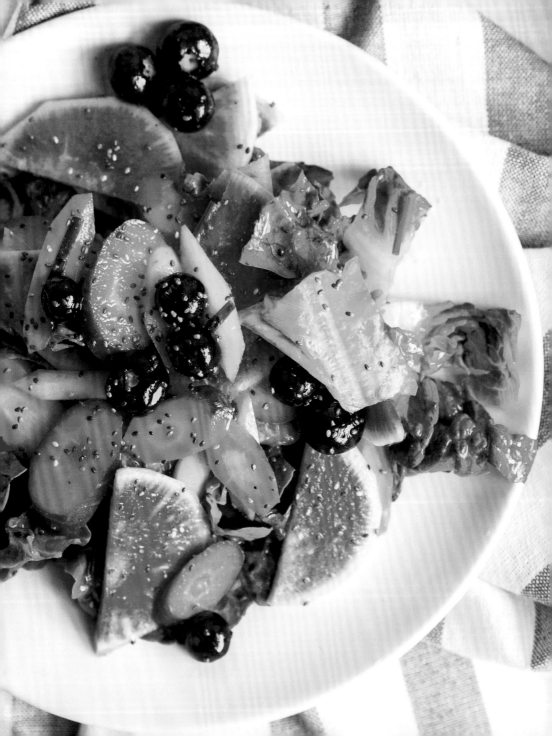

PART TWO

THE 2-WEEK PLAN TO CLEAN SKIN

So far, we've covered the **6 causes behind imperfect skin** (see pages 19–22)—inflammation, microbiome disturbance, oxidative damage, blood sugar issues, nutritional deficiencies, and hormonal imbalances—and how to address these with a more holistic, natural approach.

We've also covered the **5 skin types** —Amber, Olivia, Heath, Emmett, and Sage—and their primary root causes (see pages 23–30). Knowing which type you are is important to customizing a plan for your concerns. If you're uncertain, take my *Skin Quiz* (TheSkinQuiz.com) before proceeding.

Now let's delve into the two-week program to help you achieve clear, glowing skin naturally!

THERE ARE FOUR STEPS TO THIS 2-WEEK PROGRAM

1. Clean Plate (diet): Learn specifics on eating anti-inflammatory foods that support the liver, kidneys, and digestion, and avoid common foods that trigger skinflammation.

2. Clean Slate (toxin takeaway): Discover how to replace toxic ingredients in skin care with cleaner, effective alternatives, and follow additional recommendations to reduce toxins in the air, as well as the water and food you consume.

3. Clean Body (detox support): Stock up on herbal and nutritional supplements that boost liver and kidney function and enhance toxin removal. Take advantage of spa-cleansing techniques used for hundreds of years at spas and by naturopathic doctors.

4. Clean Mind (emotional cleansing): Evaluate emotional triggers that may have an adverse effect on the skin. When we're pushed out of our comfort zone, it's important to take this step for the body, mind, and soul—and thus the skin.

The ultimate results of this 2-week program are a clean plate, slate, body, mind . . . and glowing skin!

CHAPTER 3

Clean Plate

A clean plate is about consuming a nourishing, cleansing diet. By the end
of this chapter, you'll know the best foods for skin and why
they're so important to skin health.

It's important to see food as something we consume to nourish the body rather than simply to fill us up. My hope is that by the end of this program, your eating will become intuitive and you'll reach for these foods because you love how they make you look and feel. This journey is not about deprivation. If you follow this clean-plate step precisely, you're sure to feel rejuvenated inside and out, and enjoy the food on your plate too!

This is not a typical "cleanse" as the term has come to be understood. For those plans, some people essentially starve themselves, while others may refrain from common unhealthy habits for a week or two only to return to their SAD (standard American diet), replete with processed, imbalanced food choices. Don't think of this as a quick fix but rather as a means to reboot your diet and put your body back on a healthier path.

The daily choices we make over the long term make the biggest difference—I can't emphasize this enough. In my twenty years of studying naturopathic medicine, I've seen people yo-yo between diets and life-style choices that have a huge effect on their well-being. When you're in a healthy state, you will not do this. We all slip up—it's

normal. So don't feel guilty if (or when) it happens. But when it comes down to it, the healthy habits we stick with are the ones that feel natural and, eventually, easy. Getting there isn't always easy, so this plan is designed to help you reach the next level in your wellness journey.

A HEALTHY DIET FOR GLOWING SKIN AND VIBRANT HEALTH

We know what we eat can nourish our bodies, including the skin. The most important foods to eat for clear, glowing skin are those rich in:

▸ Skin-loving fatty acids

▸ Antioxidants

▸ Probiotics and prebiotics

▸ Collagen-boosting nutrients

▸ Cleansing and anti-inflammatory properties

These quality foods boost your body's detoxification pathways, reverse oxidative damage, and, ultimately, stop skinflammation.

Each of the following food categories includes recommended servings of a few foods known to help enhance skin.

VEGETABLES

▶ **6 or more servings per day** (see page 54 for recommended serving sizes)

Vegetables come straight from nature and are perfectly made to nurture our skin from within. Their high antioxidant, vitamin, mineral, and fiber contents make them one of the most important food groups for skin health. Most people don't eat enough vegetables. According to the U.S. Centers for Disease Control and Prevention (CDC), less than 14 percent of Americans consume the recommended amount of 2 to 3 cups (weight varies) of vegetables daily. Stop for a moment, and add up the number of vegetable servings you ate yesterday. Did you have six or more servings?

I recommend *at least 3 cups of vegetables per day*. You may be wondering how you'll fit all that in. Here's how: Eat at least 2 servings of veggies with each of your three meals, eat extras for snacks, and you've easily surpassed the recommended minimum. Choose zucchini, cucumber, and carrot slices instead of chips for a snack. Throw veggies into your morning smoothie. Eat at least one salad every day, and when you're ordering or preparing it, pile on the vegetables. Enjoy steamed veggies as a side, and include them in soups and stews. Easy! You'll find lots of veggie-packed recipes in this book to help.

"It's the daily choices we make over the long term that make the biggest difference—I can't emphasize this enough."

SKIN-NOURISHING TIPS
Include 2 to 3 servings per day of broccoli and other cruciferous veggies.

Broccoli is part of the brassica and cruciferous vegetable family. Other veggies in this family include brussels sprouts, cabbage, cauliflower, collards, kale, mustard greens, radishes, rutabaga, and turnips. They're excellent for enhancing detoxification and have a higher anticancer phytochemical content than any other vegetable family. The glucosinolates in these vegetables—in particular indole-3-carbinol, sulforaphane, diindolylmethane (DIM) and isothiocyanate—enhance antioxidant properties and improve liver detoxification. Indole-3-carbinole increases the liver's ability to metabolize estrogen by almost 50 percent.

Choose any veggie in this family if detoxification is your aim. I suggest lightly steaming these vegetables to increase nutrient absorption and remove goitrogenic properties that can suppress the thyroid gland. Broccoli is also a great source of vitamin C, biotin, and other micronutrients important for skin health.

Other skin-nourishing vegetables to enjoy include asparagus; cucumber; greens such as collard greens, kale, leeks, lettuce, and Swiss chard; onions; sea vegetables; spinach; spaghetti squash; sprouts; water chestnuts; yams; yellow squash; and zucchini.

WHAT'S IN A SERVING?

Here are my guidelines for what constitutes 1 recommended serving in each food category.

- **Vegetables:** 1 serving = ½ cup (weight varies based on vegetable) raw/uncooked vegetables

- **Fruit:**

   sweet fruit: 1 serving = 1 apple, orange, or pear; 1 cup (145 g) berries; 2 kiwis; 1 cup (150 g) watermelon cubes; 1 cup (140 g) papaya chunks; 15 cherries or grapes; 2 fresh figs; 2 apricots or plums

   savory fruit: ½ to 1 avocado, 1 to 2 tablespoons (15 to 30 ml) avocado oil, 1 to 2 tablespoons (15 to 30 ml) olive oil, or 3 to 6 olives

- **Clean animal protein:** 1 serving = 3 to 4 ounces (85 to 115 g) wild fish; grass-fed beef; wild game, such as buffalo, boar, venison, and elk; free-range chicken; and pastured pork (unless you are vegetarian for philosophical reasons; then it's 0)

- **Nuts and seeds:** 1 serving = 12 almonds or hazelnuts; 8 walnut or pecan halves; 9 cashews; 4 Brazil nuts; 3 tablespoons (15 g) coconut flesh or flakes; 1 tablespoon (16 g) nut butter; 2 tablespoons (20 g) seeds, such as pumpkin, sesame, chia, or sunflower; 2 tablespoons (8 to 9 g) pine nuts or pistachios

- **Legumes (beans and peas):** 1 serving = ½ cup (130 g) cooked beans, 1 cup (235 ml) soup, or ¼ cup (70g) bean dip

- **Gluten-free grains:** 1 serving = ½ cup (92.5 g) cooked grains, 1 slice gluten-free bread, or 1 corn-free tortilla

- **Fermented foods:** 1 serving = ½ cup (about 70 g)

- **Oils:** 1 serving = 1 tablespoon (15 ml) avocado, olive, or sesame oil; 1 tablespoon (20 g) organic virgin coconut oil

- **Herbs and spices:** servings vary, but in general 1 serving = 1 teaspoon fresh herbs and spices or ½ teaspoon dried herbs and spices

- **Liquids:** 1 serving = 8-ounce (235 ml) glass of water

STARCHY VEGETABLES

Starchy vegetables such as beets, carrots, winter squash, and yams have a high glycemic index, meaning they have a tendency to increase blood sugar. I recommend limiting your intake of these starchier veggies to 1 to 2 servings per day. They still have great value in your diet because of their high antioxidant and fiber content, so don't skip them—just don't opt for these alone when trying to meet your daily veggie intake quota.

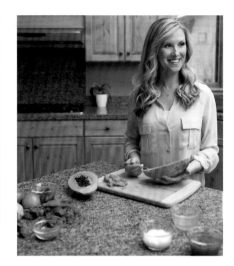

FRUIT

▸ **1 to 3 servings per day** (see page 54 for recommended serving sizes)

Fruit is rich in antioxidants, vitamins, minerals, and fiber. I suggest limiting your intake of "sweet" fruits (apples, apricots, berries, cherries, fresh figs, grapes, kiwis, oranges, pears, papayas, plums, or watermelon) due to their higher natural sugar content. When I say "sweet," I mean compared to other produce you may think of as a vegetable but that is actually a fruit, such as avocados and olives. I recommend consuming fruit in moderation because eating the "sweet" fruits in excess can increase your blood sugar. However, you still should eat fruits every day because of their high nutritional content.

If you believe your skin issues are related to glycation and blood sugar, limit your intake to 1 serving daily of "sweet" fruit. If your blood sugar is well balanced, you can enjoy 2 to 3 servings of these fruits.

In addition to "sweet" fruit, I recommend adding avocados and olives (and their oils) to your diet. While you may enjoy avocados mashed in guacamole, or indulge in olives with meat and cheese, both avocados and olives are technically classified as a fruit.

AVOCADOS

An avocado a day may just keep the dermatologist away. This soft, green fruit contains monounsaturated fats, which are "good" fats for your body, including your skin. They're high in antioxidants such as polyphenols and vitamin E, which help combat oxidative damage that can accelerate skin aging, and good fats help nourish our skin cells.

OLIVES

Olives are similar to avocados because they're not high in sugar, and they are a great source of monounsaturated fats and antioxidants. If you enjoy olives, feel free to add an extra serving to your daily fruit intake.

PAPAYAS

Papayas are rich in vitamins A and C and contain potassium, folate, fiber, and other skin-enhancing nutrients. They also naturally contain the enzyme papain, which can help us digest food. Applied topically, this fruit can also be a great exfoliator.

BERRIES

We know how important antioxidants are for skin, and these tasty treats from nature are rich in a variety of antioxidants, including flavonoids. Pick your favorite: Blackberries, blueberries, cranberries, raspberries, and strawberries are all beneficial for your skin. The ellagic acid found in berries is a powerful scavenger of superoxide radicals and can help protect cells from DNA damage. When it's hard to find fresh berries, frozen berries are a great choice because they still offer antioxidant benefits. Reach for the organic variety to reduce your pesticide exposure.

CLEAN ANIMAL PROTEIN

▶ **1 to 3 servings per day** (see page 54 for recommended serving sizes)

Animal protein provides your body with amino acids and collagen, important for healthy skin. When we eat protein, our body digests and breaks it down into amino acids, some of which are called "essential" because we can only obtain them through our diet. We need amino acids to help break down food and to grow and repair a number of other body functions, such as building muscle and healing injuries. Amino acids also help keep our skin smooth, firm, and healthy.

We also need certain amino acids to support one of the most abundant proteins in our body: collagen. As we've discussed, collagen is important for healthy skin. Consuming grass-fed beef, organic poultry, wild fish, and nuts usually provides a sufficient amount of amino acids such as arginine, glutamine, lysine, and proline—all components that can help support collagen production. We can also obtain collagen from meat when consuming tougher cuts (the tougher the meat, the higher it is in collagen), as well as skin, tendons, and bones. Later I'll explain how to make stews and bone broth to help you pick the best food sources for collagen.

CLEAN ANIMAL PROTEINS TO EAT

Number of servings per day varies (see page 54, and following, for recommended serving sizes)

Wild fish; grass-fed beef; game such as buffalo, boar, venison, and elk; free-range chicken; and pastured pork are all good choices for animal protein; but as with all things food, moderation is key! Often, serving sizes of meat are unrealistic—for your body and the planet. Keep in mind where your food comes from and what it takes to get it to your plate. Quality and quantity are both essential, and 3 to 4 ounces (85 to 115 g) per serving is all you need. If you consume too much, you negatively affect the environment—and you'll likely see skinflammation.

COLLAGEN

Collagen, a naturally occurring fibrous protein, composes 70 to 80 percent of the skin's dry weight and is the most abundant protein in the human body. It's considered the glue that holds the body together and also provides skin elasticity and strength.

You've already learned that collagen production naturally depletes as we get older, and too much sun exposure, consuming excess sugar, and smoking can expedite this process. Improving these habits is the first step to ramping up collagen production. If you've already ticked off those boxes, it's time to go a step further to combat signs of aging, such as wrinkles and sagging skin.

Many people buy topical treatments that contain collagen or undergo procedures such as skin filler injections or laser treatments that can drain our bank accounts and come with unwanted side effects. While these can affect your skin's appearance, you can get even longer-lasting benefits by being more cognizant of what you put in your body.

A NOTE ON COOKING MEAT

I know we love to barbecue, but if you want a glowing complexion, limit barbecued meats. At temperatures above 248°F (120°C), sugars bind to proteins to form AGEs. Cooking foods at high temperatures—such as barbecuing—increases AGEs. Research has linked eating meat cooked at high temperatures with certain cancers. You don't have to avoid barbecuing, but limit your barbecue time and throw veggies on the grill too. They'll help you meet your daily target veggie intake, and barbecuing them does not have the same potentially harmful effect as with high-heat-cooked meat.

The number of servings of animal protein you should eat depends upon any nutritional deficiencies you have, your height and weight, and how many other non-animal protein servings you consume. If you are small framed and eat a few servings of legumes and nuts every day, you may only need 1 or 2 servings of animal protein. If you struggle with eating legumes or nuts and have a large stature, you will need 2 or 3 servings of animal protein per day while you adjust to eating more non-animal protein sources.

MY FAVORITE SKIN-NOURISHING ANIMAL PROTEIN

I've said this before: Wild salmon is rich in omega-3s, which possess anti-inflammatory properties. Because the root of many skin problems is inflammation, this is one of the most important nutrients for skin health. Salmon's pink color indicates it contains the antioxidant astaxanthin, which studies suggest has sun-protective effects and can counteract UVA-induced skin changes. Whenever you have a choice between farmed and wild-caught salmon, *always* opt for wild. Farmed salmon does not contain the same amount of beneficial omega-3s and contains more environmental contaminants.

BUT I'M A VEGAN

If you have philosophical, religious, or personal reasons for not eating meat, then follow this program as a vegan. Consider, though, that there are certain nutrients crucial for skin that we cannot obtain as easily when eating a vegan diet. (I say vegan because you'll avoid eggs and dairy on this program.) While it's true that vegetables, grains, legumes, and nuts do contain protein and other important nutrients, you will need to look elsewhere to get the crucial nutrients that meat can provide. Meat is a great source of amino acids, iron, vitamin B12, and zinc, which are essential nutrients for skin health. If you're vegan, I strongly recommend taking supplements.

NUTS AND SEEDS

▸ **1 to 2 servings per day** (see page 54 for recommended serving sizes)

Nuts and seeds possess essential fatty acids, minerals, vitamin E, and protein—but avoid nuts coated with salt or crusted with honey and sugar. Choose whole, organic, high-quality nuts. Eat nuts and seeds every day, but don't go overboard. Most people only need 1 to 2 servings per day.

It's best to get nuts in the shell and crack them open, but this can be inconvenient. When choosing shelled nuts, choose whole nuts because the chopped, sliced, and broken nuts are more likely to be rancid (when the oils oxidize and go "bad"). Store shelled nuts in airtight containers and use them quickly. If they smell as though they've gone bad, throw them out.

Nuts are a great food, but NOT if you're allergic to them! Nuts are one of the top food allergens, causing reactions that can be severe and, for some people, life threatening. More than 1 percent of Americans have a tree nut and peanut allergy, and that number is on the rise. A 2013 report by the *World Allergy Organization Journal* notes that the prevalence of food allergies in preschool children in developed countries is now as high as 10 percent, with the prevalence, severity, and complexity of food allergies increasing in both developed and developing nations.

You likely know whether you have an allergy; if you're not sure, though, see an allergy specialist to be tested. Cashews are part of the mango and pistachio family, so if you have allergies to one of these, you likely will react to all three. Seeds such as pumpkin (pepitas), flax, sunflower, and sesame are well tolerated in some people who have nut allergies.

Fungi can grow on certain types of nuts that are low quality and have been improperly stored (in warm, humid places). The FDA has rules to help protect us, but it is best to choose nuts from a grocery store you know stores them in a cool, dry environment.

Roasting is thought to protect the nuts against fungi growth, but roasting can actually oxidize the nut oils so they are no longer beneficial. Not to mention, most commercial roasting involves deep-frying (not good for skin)!

Nuts are high in a number of amino acids, including arginine. While this amino acid is important, a diet high in arginine can trigger cold sores or herpes virus infections in susceptible people. In our bodies there is a lysine (another amino acid) and arginine balance. When this is thrown off, people with herpes are more likely to suffer an outbreak. If you're prone to cold sores or herpes and feel you have an outbreak coming on, decrease your nut intake to 1 serving per day and take a lysine supplement.

MY FAVORITE NUT

Coconut! Enjoy the whole coconut. There are benefits from the water, milk, meat, and oil this precious plant produces. Coconut contains lauric acid, also found in human breast milk, which is full of immune-enhancing properties that are great for skin health. Our bodies convert lauric acid to monolaurin, which has antimicrobial effects, fighting viruses, bacteria, and other infectious microorganisms. Consuming coconut may help reduce the frequency of breakouts and skin infections, as well as keep our skin healthy from the inside out. There also are great benefits of the oil.

LEGUMES (BEANS AND PEAS)

▸ **1 to 3 servings per day** (see page 54 for recommended serving sizes)

Legumes (beans and peas) contain important nutrients, are great sources of fiber and protein, and can help balance blood sugar. All of these qualities make legumes a top skin-nourishing food. The colorful red, black, pinto, and kidney beans are all rich in antioxidants. In fact, red kidney beans have a higher antioxidant content than blueberries! In addition to antioxidants, beans are high in folic acid, vitamin B6, magnesium, iron, manganese, and potassium. Peas, including garden, sugar snap, and snow varieties, all contain similar nutritional qualities to beans.

If you are vegan or vegetarian, I recommend consuming 3 servings of legumes per day. If you're an omnivore, consume 1 to 2 servings daily. To get more legumes in your diet, eat peas, lentils, hummus, and an array of colorful beans. Dips, soups, or salads containing legumes are a creative and tasty way to eat even more. You've probably heard the old saying, "Beans, beans, the magical fruit. The more you eat the more you toot." Well, they're not a fruit, but they are magical and, for some people, do create gas. That's because

SOAKING NUTS AND SEEDS

Soaking activates and increases nutrients such as vitamins A, B, and C; inactivates enzyme inhibitors; and makes foods such as nuts, grains, and legumes easier to digest.

HOW TO SOAK NUTS AND SEEDS

You can use these nutrient-filled soaked nuts and seeds as skin-healthy snacks or to make plant-based milk alternatives or nut butters. They're also great added to salads and smoothies.

1. Place the raw nuts or seeds in a large glass bowl or jar and cover with filtered water (about twice as much water as nuts).

2. Add ¼ to ½ teaspoon Himalayan salt or Celtic sea salt. Cover with a light cloth and set aside to soak overnight.

3. Drain and rinse the nuts or seeds thoroughly; keep refrigerated.

they contain oligosaccharides, which the body doesn't digest; they travel along to the intestines, where bacteria break them down and create gas as a by-product. You can reduce the amount of oligosaccharides (and gas) by properly preparing beans for consumption (see page 60).

TIPS ON PREPARING LEGUMES

Whether you eat legumes regularly or they're new to you, I encourage you to eat at least 1 serving daily to reap their skin-healthy benefits.

SOAKING

Soak beans, covered with a few inches of filtered water, overnight in your refrigerator. For lentils, I recommend soaking for 15 minutes to 1 hour before cooking. Soaking helps reduce the cooking time and helps your body enjoy their benefits more easily.

Rinse the soaked beans to remove the sudsy-looking water or any skins that have floated to the surface. Do not add seasoning or salt until after the beans are cooked. Depending upon the type, legumes can take anywhere from 30 minutes to 3 hours to cook. Refer to the package instructions for cooking times. If you're strapped for time, use cooked beans in recipes, or as a side dish. If purchasing canned foods, however, look for BPA-free cans. This chemical, used in the lining of many food cans, has hormone-disrupting effects.

SPROUTING

Because legumes are seeds, you can sprout them, which increases their nutritional content and makes them easier to digest. To sprout beans, rinse them, place them in an open jar, cover with warm filtered water, and set aside for 24 hours. Rinse and refill the water several times during this period. Most beans will sprout and be ready to eat after 1 or 2 days.

GLUTEN-FREE GRAINS

▸ **0 to 1 serving per day** (see page 54 for recommended serving sizes)

Grains are a good source of fiber, minerals, and certain B vitamins. While whole grains are considered "healthy," most people eat too many in the form of bagels, rolls, sandwich bread, cereals, etc. With this kind of diet, we consume excessive amounts of the most common grains: wheat and corn. The high demand has led the food industry to increase production by genetically modifying these grains. These alterations are not healthy for our bodies, and many health experts believe there is a connection between a rise in sensitivities and allergies to these modified grains and their overconsumption. Excessive intake also can lead to blood sugar regulation problems.

To obtain the benefits of grains without their potential drawbacks, as part of my two-week program, I recommend eating only 1 serving of gluten- and corn-free whole grains, such as quinoa and rice. You can also go entirely grain free during the two-week program. You will still obtain all the nutrients, including fiber, from the other aspects of the program. If you do choose to eat grains, consider eating them as a side dish accompanying a protein and vegetables, and limit your servings.

Many people think "gluten free" makes grains a healthy choice. Unfortunately, with the increased popularity of gluten-free eating, food companies are mass-producing these foods, and many have lost sight of the quality of ingredients. Check your ingredient labels. You will likely find sugar and other sweeteners as well as heavily processed ingredients in these gluten-free items. It's usually best to make your own gluten-free product unless you have a trusted source.

MY FAVORITE GRAIN

Quinoa is a gluten-free, protein-rich grain. It is very satiating, in part due to its high protein and amino acid content. You can make it into a nice, warm breakfast similar to oatmeal or serve it warm as a side dish or cold as a salad.

Other gluten-free grain options include amaranth, brown or red rice, buckwheat, millet, and gluten-free oats.

Yes, oats can be gluten free. This skin-nourishing food is packed with fiber and nutrients (B_1, manganese, and selenium) because the hulling process doesn't strip away the bran and germ as is the case for more-processed grains. What's more, the fiber in oats contains high amounts of beta-glucan, which can help lower cholesterol. But because oats have a higher fat content than other grains, the oils can go rancid more easily. Buy oats in small quantities, and use them by the recommended date on the packaging. If the grain smells bad, throw it out. Also, although oats are gluten free, they are also one of the more common food allergens.

Rice has high fiber content, but it contains less protein than whole wheat. Brown rice can go rancid fairly easily, so it's best to keep it refrigerated once you open it.

WHY WE WANT WHOLE GRAINS, NOT PROCESSED GRAINS

The process of refining grains removes the bran and germ, which in turn removes certain nutrients. To make up for this, processed, or white, flours are "enriched" to add nutrients back in. I prefer nature's version—the whole form. Whole grains are higher in fiber, protein, and nutrients. Refined grains also contain chemicals from the refining and bleaching process.

Amaranth is a lesser-known grain that's gluten free, rich in nutrients, and has a high protein and fiber content (having more fiber than whole wheat!). Compared with other grains, amaranth is much less allergenic. However, it's hard to find foods made strictly from amaranth—commonly you'll find it in a combination multigrain product.

Buckwheat contains high-quality protein, flavonoids, and fiber.

Millet is a tiny bead-shaped grain with higher protein content than corn, wheat, and rice. You can use millet as a breakfast cereal or ground as part of gluten-free multigrain flour. Millet contains goitrogen, which interferes with thyroid function, so people with hypothyroidism should not consume millet every day. Sometimes this grain is not well tolerated by individuals with celiac disease, despite the fact it is gluten free.

I believe these whole grains, when properly prepared and consumed in moderation, are a healthy and satisfying option for our palates and skin.

FERMENTED FOODS

▸ **1 to 2 servings per day** (see page 54 for recommended serving sizes)

Fermented vegetables, such as sauerkraut and coconut yogurt, are good food sources of probiotics, which we know support the growth and maintenance of friendly bacteria, such as *Lactobacillus acidophilus* and bifidobacteria.

If you are new to these foods, start with 1 serving per day. As your body adjusts to the beneficial microorganisms, you may experience mild gas and bloating. This should subside within a few days; if it doesn't, you may need additional digestive and microbiome support. If you already consume these foods regularly, eat 1 or 2 servings daily to enhance your gut and skin health. As always, choose the highest-quality foods or, ideally, make your own. I include a few recipes for probiotic-rich meals and drinks, and there are many more available. When making your own, follow the directions carefully so you grow only the right (good) kinds of bacteria.

OILS

▸ Daily servings vary depending on how much animal protein, nuts, avocados, olives, and other fat-containing foods you consume. **If you eat the recommended amounts of each food, you should consume an extra 4 to 6 servings per day of oils** (see page 54 for recommended serving sizes).

Some of the most skin-enriching oils come from coconut, sesame seeds, avocado, and olives. These are antioxidant rich, with nutrients such as vitamins E and A. Olive oil is a component of the Mediterranean diet, which has been shown to be anti-inflammatory; it's my favorite choice for salad dressings and garnishing food after cooking.

It's best to choose unrefined, cold-pressed oils. Many oils are made by chemical extraction using a chemical solvent that separates the oil, which is then exposed to high heat and additional chemicals. Traces of the chemical solvents may remain, and refining oils remove their nutrients.

I love coconut oil for cooking because it's stable at high temperatures and not as susceptible to oxidative damage from heat as olive oil and vegetable oils. Plus, coconut oils are good sources of fats for our skin. Use it in baking or cooking, but keep in mind it does impart a coconut flavor. Personally, I think it's yummy, but it doesn't go well in everything. If you don't want the flavor of coconut in whatever you're cooking or baking, avocado oil is a nice alternative.

HERBS AND SPICES

▸ **At least 2 serving per day** (see page 54 for recommended serving sizes)

There are numerous and delicious antioxidant-rich, anti-inflammatory herbs great for skin and overall health. Here are some of my favorites for both their health properties and their flavor.

▸ Cilantro (coriander leaf): high in vitamins K and A

▸ Cinnamon: aids digestion; improves circulation

▸ Cumin: helps liver detoxification; aids digestion

▸ Fennel: aids digestion

▸ Fennel seed: aids digestion

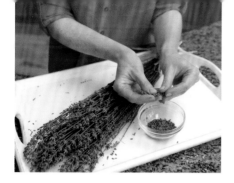

- Garlic: Its pungent aroma is from allicin, a sulfur compound, released when garlic is cut or crushed; it also has great anti-microbial properties and is well known for its health benefits.

- Ginger: aids digestion

- Parsley: rich in vitamin C

- Rosemary: rich in antioxidants and has anti-inflammatory properties; aids digestion

- Thyme: rich in antioxidants, with anti-inflammatory and antimicrobial properties

- Turmeric: rich in anti-inflammatory and antioxidant properties; helps liver detoxification

LIQUIDS

- **6 or more servings per day** (see page 54 for recommended serving sizes)

Filtered water should be your primary drink. I recommend starting every morning with an 8-ounce (235 ml) glass of filtered water, because when you sleep, your body is deprived of hydration. When you wake from a full night's rest, your body will have been without water for six to eight hours. If you think "plain" water is unappetizing, try "spa water:" Fill a large pitcher with filtered water and add cucumber slices; fresh berries; or orange, lemon, or lime slices.

If you consume other beverages, drink at least four glasses of filtered water plus two or more of the following:

- Sparkling water is a nice treat if you're used to sodas or want something a bit more exciting. You can "spice" it up with some "spa water."

- Herbal tea is a great option for additional hydration. Keep in mind that some herbal teas have diuretic properties; you may notice the need to urinate more, and your urine may appear clearer than usual. That's okay, but be sure to drink filtered water as well. It's best to limit herbal tea consumption to 1 to 4 cups daily. Some of my favorites for their health-promoting benefits are:

Burdock root	Chamomile
Chicory	Dandelion
Fennel	Milk thistle
Rooibos	Yellow dock

- Fresh coconut water from green coconuts contains antioxidants that are super hydrating. You can buy coconut water in stores, but limit consumption to 8 ounces (235 ml) per day because of the high natural sugar content, and make sure there are no other ingredients or added sugar. Choose fresh when possible.

- Smoothies can be a great drink or snack. See chapter 7 for recipes and information.

- Bone broth is full of collagen, which is crucial for reducing fine lines and wrinkles. Use only bones from organic animals. For extra collagen, you can add gelatin. It may be an adventurous choice, but the benefits of bone broth and gelatin are huge. See chapter 8 for recipes.

MEAL TIMING AND OTHER DIETARY CONSIDERATIONS

Before you start the two-week program, I highly recommend you do some menu planning and create a schedule. I do *not* want you to skip any meals. This is not a fast.

Eat three meals daily (breakfast, lunch, and dinner), plus one or two snacks. Although some people drop excess fat during this program, this is not a weight-loss plan.

Here is how to schedule your meals, which will vary depending on your schedule:

Eat breakfast within 1 hour of waking. If you wake before 9 a.m., have a mid-morning snack three to four hours later. Eat lunch three to four hours after that, followed by a mid-afternoon snack three to four hours later. If you eat dinner before

A NOTE ON EXERCISE AND EATING

If you start your morning with a smoothie, you may be able to exercise one hour later. If you have digestive issues or eat a large breakfast, you may need to wait two hours or longer before exercising. It's important not to exercise in the morning without first consuming at least a smoothie. You've been fasting overnight, and your body needs fuel. It's also good to eat a snack or meal after exercising to ensure your body has the necessary nutrients for recovery.

6 p.m., skip the mid-afternoon snack. Do not eat within two hours of bedtime. For example:

Wake	6 a.m.
Breakfast	6:30 a.m. (within 1 hour of waking)
Snack	9:30 a.m. (3 to 4 hours after breakfast)
Lunch	12:30 p.m. (3 to 4 hours after mid-morning snack)
Snack	3:30 p.m. (3 to 4 hours after lunch)
Dinner	6:30 p.m. (do not eat within 1 to 2 hours of bedtime)
Bedtime	10 p.m.

FOODS TO ELIMINATE ON THE 2-WEEK PROGRAM

While there are foods that make your skin glow, there are others that tend to trigger inflammation. These foods aren't "bad," but I suggest you eliminate them for at least fourteen days.

Here are ten foods (and their family members)—in order of importance—to eliminate. I've found sugar and dairy to be the most significant skinflammation triggers.

1. Sugar (agave syrup, cane sugar, corn syrup, high-fructose corn syrup, sugar)

2. Dairy (cheese, cottage cheese, ice cream, milk, yogurt, etc.)

3. Gluten-containing grains (spelt, wheat, etc.)

4. Alcohol (beer, liquor, wine, etc.)

5. Caffeine (chocolate, coffee, tea, soda)

6. Eggs (whites and yolks from any bird)

7. Corn (corn chips, kernels, popcorn, etc.)

8. Nightshades (eggplant, goji berries, peppers, potatoes, tomatoes, and tomatillos)

9. Peanuts (peanut butter, peanuts [raw or roasted])

10. Soy (edamame, soy milk, tofu, etc.)

Also eliminate any processed or artificial ingredients—colors, flavor enhancers, sweeteners, HFCS, hydrogenated oils, and vegetable oils. I recommend avoiding these foods even when you're not on the program.

Again, these are not "bad" foods, and not all these foods may trigger problems for you. The idea is to give up these foods for fourteen days to see how your skin fares without them in your diet. You'll then have the opportunity to reintroduce some, or all, of these foods and evaluate whether any create issues for you. Let's look at each of the ten foods individually.

COMMON SUGAR SUBSTITUTES

▸ Honey: although natural, it affects blood sugar (avoid or use in small amounts)

▸ Maple syrup: a natural sweetener that affects blood sugar (avoid or use in small amounts)

▸ Stevia: a natural plant sweetener (*my favorite*) that does not affect blood sugar

▸ Xylitol or erythritol: a sugar alcohol that does not affect blood sugar

SUGAR

Americans eat an average of 22.2 teaspoons (88.8 g) of sugar per day—a shockingly large amount that can increase the risk of fatty liver disease, type 2 diabetes, kidney disease, obesity, and skin problems. Aside from candy, cookies, and cakes, sugar also lurks in unexpected places, such as bread, salad dressings, and tomato sauce. Research suggests sugar is highly addictive due to its strong effect on the brain's reward center. According to a paper published in the journal *PLOS ONE* in 2007, rats chose sugar over cocaine when they had a choice because the sugar reward is stronger.

We know sugar is particularly bad for skin. Its highly acidic nature throws off the delicate pH within the body, and it is a pro-inflammatory food. Also, eating sugar increases blood glucose, which increases insulin; and because high insulin has been shown to stimulate sebum production and androgen activity, it can trigger acne.

As we've discussed, sugar increases glycation's collagen-damaging effects and accelerates skin's aging.

If you eat sugar regularly, reduce consumption gradually. Switch to honey and maple syrup for a few days leading up to the two-week program. After a few days, most people don't miss sugar.

DAIRY

Dairy is a problem food group for skin, and studies suggest skim milk can be especially harmful. Dairy is pro-inflammatory and a common food allergen. In addition, there are hormones in dairy. Milk from cows that are not given hormones contains natural growth hormones and anabolic steroids to help calves grow. Even if you buy "hormone-free" dairy products, bypassing all hormones in dairy is nearly impossible. Consuming hormones can create imbalances when they interact with the body's natural hormones.

Lactose, found in milk, has a high sugar content, which we know increases the potential for skin damage. A study published in the May 2008 issue of the *Journal of the American Academy of Dermatology* suggested a closer correlation between skim milk and acne compared with other types of dairy.

Does this mean you can never eat dairy again? No! There's a good chance you can find a balance after the two-week program with some dairy consumption in easier-to-digest forms, such as yogurt and certain cheeses.

GLUTEN

Whether whole grains or refined, gluten appears to be a trigger food for many people with skin conditions. Some people erupt with exposure to just a dusting of flour, while other people's skin problems emerge when gluten is consumed in excess. Avoiding gluten can prove challenging, as the standard American diet includes gluten-laden cereals and pastries for breakfast; sandwiches for lunch; and pasta, bread, or breaded foods at dinnertime—not to mention gluten-packed snacks and desserts. And with many of these choices, you get the combo of high sugar, which can lead to glycation issues. Gluten is one of the top allergenic foods that contribute to skin inflammation issues.

Emerging research shows gluten is not just a problem for those with celiac disease. Dermatitis herpetiformis, for example, is strongly linked to a gluten reaction. Studies also suggest a link between gluten intolerance and skin conditions such as eczema, psoriasis, and vitiligo.

As we've discussed, there are other reactions to gluten besides celiac disease, such as IgG and IgA, also known as "intolerances" or "sensitivities." For people who are gluten reactive, eating gluten can increase the digestive tract lining's permeability. This allows proteins to cross the lining and get into your bloodstream. Your immune system

---

SOME DAIRY ALTERNATIVES

There are many more options available than what I've listed here. Check the ingredient labels to ensure the foods do not have "hidden" sugar or other ingredients on the "foods to avoid" list.

- ▸ Almond, hazelnut, and hemp milks
- ▸ Coconut oil (instead of butter)
- ▸ Coconut (unsweetened)
- ▸ Unsweetened coconut and almond yogurts

goes into overdrive and increases inflammation, which can trigger acne and other skin issues. We've also learned that foods with a high glycemic index, such as pastries, breads, and pastas, cause blood sugar and insulin to spike, triggering acne.

Is gluten an acne trigger for everyone? I don't think so, but I do find it is for many. Simply switching to gluten-free grains does not solve the problem. All grains, when consumed in excess or without balancing with adequate dietary proteins, can increase blood sugar, insulin, and sebum production—and therefore trigger acne breakouts. That's why limiting daily grain intake is so important.

ALCOHOL

Alcohol is high in sugar and can dehydrate the body, so it is not a good choice for a skin-healthy diet. In addition, alcohol is tough on our livers and depletes our bodies of important nutrients. I recommend taking a break from alcohol during the two-week program. Afterward, you may find a happy balance. We'll discuss this further in chapter 10.

People often ask me, "What about red wine?" Red wine does contain the antioxidant resveratrol, and some research suggests a link between regular, moderate consumption of alcohol and a reduced risk for heart disease. There are many other ways to obtain antioxidants (including resveratrol) and promote heart health—and those options don't pose the health harms that alcohol can. If you are a Heath-type (see pages 26–27), this is particularly important for you, as alcohol is a trigger for inflammatory conditions such as rosacea.

TIPS TO ELIMINATE CAFFEINE

If, after trying these tips, you still have headaches, or you can't bear the thought of going two weeks without caffeine, that's usually a sign you're addicted to it. If you "can't live without caffeine," sip 1 cup of green tea per day for its great skin-protecting effects.

▸ Taper off for a few days before the program by reducing your daily amount by ½ cup (120 ml).

▸ If you begin suffering from headaches or nausea, drink weak black or green tea.

▸ Do not overindulge before or after the caffeine cleanse.

CAFFEINE

Caffeine is dehydrating and acidic, and it can deplete certain skin-enhancing vitamins and minerals; it is not a skin-nourishing choice. Caffeine is also a nervous system stimulant that causes our body to shift into the sympathetic dominant, fight or flight mode. Because of the induced stress state, caffeine is taxing on our adrenals and neurologic system.

I will cover how you may be able to consume caffeine in moderation after the two-week program (see pages 194–195). For now, it's important to eliminate caffeine during the program to give your body a break.

EGGS

Eggs are typically thought of as a superfood. They are a good source of protein and full of B vitamins. But eggs also are one of the most common allergens (the second-most common behind dairy), and when it comes to skin, I've found eggs to be a common trigger food.

It's best to avoid them for fourteen days and see how your skin fares. I have seen a strong link between eggs consumption and both eczema (atopic dermatitis) and acne in many of my patients.

Avoid both egg whites and egg yolks; they both are food triggers leading to skinflammation. If you're skeptical, give it a try—you won't know for sure until you do. It's one trigger I see frequently, and it's often the missing piece when people have tried other elimination diets but continue to eat eggs.

CORN

Corn is a grain, not a vegetable. While corn is gluten free, it is still one of the most common food allergens. This may be partly because corn is one of the most commonly genetically modified crops. Corn is the most-produced grain in the world, in large part due to its high consumption across the globe. You may not even be aware of it, but if you read the labels of packaged foods, you'll see corn everywhere—corn syrup, high-fructose corn syrup, cornstarch, corn meal, corn flour, hydrolyzed corn, and even some artificial flavors. In other words, corn is not just found in corn bread and corn chips. It's in the majority of sodas and processed foods sold in the United Sates. Remember, it's just two weeks. I'll share how you can reintroduce corn in a healthy way afterward so that you'll know whether it's a problem food for you.

NIGHTSHADES

Nightshade fruits and vegetables (see page 65) belong to the Solanaceae plant family. Some people have a sensitivity to nightshade plants and have difficulty digesting them. If you have this food sensitivity, you may experience a number of symptoms, including gas, bloating, nausea, painful joints, headaches, moodiness, and skin issues. If you're 100 percent sure you don't have a nightshade sensitivity, skip this section. However, if you've never gone fourteen days without this family of foods, I highly recommend avoiding them to see how your skin fares. These are another one of the big "aha" foods for people who have tried elimination diets but did not see their skin clear up.

PEANUTS

Peanuts are actually a legume, not a nut, and they're one of the top food allergens. You probably know someone with a peanut allergy or are aware of the strict "peanut free" policies many schools implement today. *Aspergillus flavus* is a fungus that grows on peanuts and produces aflatoxin, which is toxic to our livers and a known carcinogen. It's best to give up peanuts during the two-week program to ensure you're not exposed to this common trigger food.

SOY

Soy has gone from being unimportant to being important and then to being labeled as dangerous. What's the truth? Soy actually isn't that bad. Like other legumes, it has a high protein and fiber content. Soy has phytoestrogens that can be helpful for perimenopausal women, yet there are concerns about effects for other people, such as those with thyroid disease, or even men and young women. The biggest problems with soy are that it is typically genetically modified and is a top allergen. It's best to avoid soy during the two-week program; then we can discuss whether this is a food to reintroduce later.

PROCESSED FOODS

While not one of the ten foods listed to avoid, popular processed foods are not good for our skin. One main reason is that most contain hydrogenated oils. Packaged foods, such as chips, are processed at high temperatures, and the oils oxidize during this process, which can increase inflammation and spur oxidative damage.

PROCESSED FOODS WITH HYDROGENATED AND VEGETABLE OILS

Hydrogenated, partially hydrogenated, and other processed oils are unnatural, contain toxic byproducts, and harm cellular membrane function.

People are more aware of the concerns over hydrogenated, or trans, fats, but many continue to cook and bake with vegetable oil. In the 1960s through the 1980s, persuasive marketing campaigns led consumers to choose vegetable oils, such as canola oil, as a staple food. However, we now know common vegetable oil is one of the worst foods for our skin. In addition to being genetically modified and highly processed, it is a source of omega-6 oils, which lead to an imbalance of the essential omega-3 to omega-6 ratio. This can lead to inflammation, reversing the good effect omega-3s have on skin.

These oils are commonly used in fast foods, which is one reason this greasy fare is bad for our skin. High-temperature heating used for fried foods oxidizes oils and creates free radical damage. It's much better to bake or steam food than to fry it. Some studies have shown that eating fried foods increases the risk for type 2 diabetes; other studies have suggested a link between consuming fried foods and developing cancer.

PROCESSED FOODS WITH HIGH-FRUCTOSE CORN SYRUP (HFCS)

HFCS is another common ingredient in processed foods and beverages. While we now know the harmful effects of this ingredient, many Americans still consume it regularly, which is contributing to the skyrocketing rates of obesity, type 2 diabetes, and fatty liver disease. High-fructose corn syrup is rapidly absorbed and quickly increases blood sugar, which leads to various internal health problems that the skin subsequently reflects. Other countries avoid HFCS in their processed foods; unfortunately the United States is still behind on this.

Though some manufacturers are slowly starting to phase out their use of HFCS, many sodas still contain the ingredient, and its caramel color is linked to an increased risk of carcinogen exposure. Dark-colored sodas are one of the worst culprits—and don't think diet sodas are better than regular. Diet sodas come with a whole host of problems despite their lower-calorie label. Studies suggest artificial sweeteners trick the body into thinking it's had something sweet, so you end up craving more sweets, eating more, and gaining weight.

Before you trade your soda for another beverage, such as fruit juice, look at the sugar level. You may be surprised to see that orange juice and bottled smoothies can have just as much, if not more, sugar than sodas. Skip those processed choices and opt for good, old-fashioned filtered water—it's the best beverage to promote skin health.

TIPS FOR SUCCESS

- Family and friends (and their homes), going out to eat, even your own home, can be triggers for unhealthy habits.

- When attending parties, bring your own food (see recipes in chapters 7 and 8). Tell the host you want to help by bringing a dish to share—at least you'll have one thing to eat.

- If you are hosting a party, serve foods that are gluten, dairy, and sugar free.

- Find an alternative drink to soda or fruit juice to cut back on sugar intake.

- Drink sparkling water (or soda water) with lime or lemon.

- Enjoy herbal teas instead of coffee.

- Need sweetness? Add a little stevia.

- Ordering appetizers? Choose a salad.

- If you're at a buffet, fill half your plate with veggies.

- Order whole foods: meat, rice, legumes, salads; stay away from casseroles and other "complicated" main courses.

- Choose restaurants that offer healthy options and will accommodate special requests.

- Prepare ahead: After grocery shopping, chop carrots, cucumbers, zucchini, and other veggies so they're easier to grab than chips or crackers.

- Skip the sandwich or pasta. Instead use salad as your base. Add veggies, beans, peas, sunflower seeds, pumpkin seeds, clean protein, and any other items on your "foods to eat" list you want.

IN SUMMARY

For two weeks, avoid the ten foods discussed—plus processed foods—because of their pro-inflammatory and gut-disturbing effects. Additionally:

- Choose whole, unprocessed, organic foods to ensure you get the highest quality, most nutrient-rich foods possible.

- Drink plenty of filtered water and herbal teas (dandelion, chicory, and milk thistle) that support kidney and liver function.

- Eat an antioxidant-rich diet, including staples such as green tea, colorful fruits and vegetables, and legumes. These help ward off free radical damage from AGEs and reduce the risk of premature aging.

- Eat 6 or more servings of vegetables per day and a couple servings of antioxidant-rich fruit. Include at least 1 daily serving of onions, garlic, and another of the brassica family, such as broccoli, cabbage, cauliflower, and brussels sprouts.

- Consume healthy oils for their anti-inflammatory omega-3s; use olive oil in salad dressings and coconut oil for cooking.

- Avoid sugar and high-carbohydrate processed foods to keep blood sugar balanced.

- Start the day with a smoothie.

- Eat balanced snacks and meals. In other words, do not eat fruits and grains without completing your plate with protein and fat.

- Add spices and herbs such as oregano, cinnamon, cloves, ginger, and garlic to your cuisine. Research shows these herbs can help stop the production of AGEs.

Most people notice a significant transformation within two weeks. If you notice only minor changes, it's a sign you're moving in the right direction and should continue on the program for another two weeks.

SYMPTOM CHECKLIST

Check off each of the following symptoms you have. Give yourself 1 point for each and then total all points at the bottom. Do this before you start the two-week program.

- □ acne
- □ dry skin
- □ rosacea
- □ eczema
- □ dermatitis
- □ psoriasis
- □ other skin rashes/eruptions
- □ skin itching
- □ fatigue
- □ lack of drive
- □ lightheadedness
- □ abdominal bloating
- □ constipation
- □ diarrhea
- □ heartburn
- □ unformed or loose stools
- □ gassiness
- □ bad breath
- □ body odor
- □ headaches
- □ migraines
- □ runny nose

- □ itchy eyes
- □ itchy nose
- □ sneezing
- □ coughing
- □ ringing in the ears
- □ body aches
- □ PMS
- □ irregular menstrual cycles
- □ painful menses
- □ irritability
- □ mood swings
- □ brain fog
- □ difficulty focusing/concentrating
- □ blurry vision
- □ weight (fat) gain
- □ inability to lose weight (fat)
- □ muscle pain
- □ joint pain
- □ other inflammatory conditions/ diseases

TOTAL POINTS: _____

CHAPTER 4

Clean Slate

Okay. You've established your clean plate. The next step is creating a clean slate. This means using products free from toxic inflammatory agents and, instead, packed with key nourishing ingredients. This is important for all skin types, particularly for those who identify with Olivia, Heath, and Emmett (see pages 25–28).

The first step to a clean slate involves taking a closer look at what you're putting on your skin. Do you know what you expose your body to every day during morning and nighttime cleansing and beauty regimens? Often, when I talk to people about giving up their regular skin care products, they resist. I get it. But pay attention to this section. It contains some of the most important information in the book.

For women, who on average tend to use more products than men, this is crucial. But, men, this applies to you too if you use deodorant, shampoo, and shaving cream.

It's important to know there are alternative ingredients that often prove healthier and less risky than those commonly used in commercial lines. So don't think you have to toss everything you own and abandon your current hygiene routine completely. After years of one-on-one counseling with clients who found these everyday products troublesome, I can tell you with confidence that natural approaches to skin care can be even *more effective* than what most people currently use.

In this chapter, I share the *true science of natural beauty*, which debunks the popular myth that natural skin care isn't effective. First, let's understand the problem with everyday skin care products.

THE DARK SIDE OF SKIN CARE

Would you slather gasoline or diesel fuel on your face? Liquid plastic, formaldehyde, or tar? Of course not! But if you're using most popular skin care products (or even some so-called "natural" skin care), there's a chance you're applying shocking ingredients like these to your face. These potentially toxic components are often hidden on skin care product labels, and most people don't know where or how to look for them. Here you'll learn just how to do that.

According to the Environmental Working Group (EWG), the average person uses nine personal care products every day, which exposes us to 126 unique ingredients. The National Institute of Occupational Safety and Health reported nearly 900 *toxic* chemicals are used in skin care and cosmetic products. While that may seem like a lot, the European Union has actually banned more than 1,000 ingredients from personal care products. Here's the kicker: The U.S. Food and Drug Administration has banned only eleven ingredients in personal care products!

This is a problem because many skin care products contain petroleum by-products, ingredients in plastics and rubber, formaldehyde-releasing chemicals, and other toxins. These are known hormone disruptors and carcinogens. While manufacturers in the United States, and the FDA itself, may claim these ingredients are safe in small amounts, the information we have does not actually support that idea. Because we're already exposed to so many toxins in our environment, why add fuel to the fire?

FIVE COMMON SKIN CARE PRODUCT INGREDIENTS TO AVOID

It's really up to you, the consumer, to be proactive about what you put in your bathroom cabinets, and on your face, and thus in your system overall. Read on to learn more about the five skin care product ingredients you should avoid.

#1 INGREDIENT TO AVOID: FRAGRANCE

This ingredient is a big one because we like to smell good, and manufacturers know that. The problem is, most skin care products contain synthetic fragrance; unfortunately, it's this ingredient wherein other potentially harmful ingredients may hide. Research reported from May 2010 by the EWG and the Campaign for Safe Cosmetics found an average of fourteen chemicals in seventeen brand-name fragrance products—*none of which were listed on the label.*

Fragrances can contain a number of endocrine disrupting chemicals (EDCs) and are among the top five allergens in the world. As discussed previously, EDCs are a class of chemicals that research has associated with certain conditions, such as thyroid problems, infertility, early menopause, early puberty, obesity, diabetes, and certain types of cancer, including prostate, testicular, and breast cancer.

One chemical of particular concern is diethyl phthalate (DEP), which is used to make plastics then used in automobile parts, toys, tools, and to make food packaging more flexible. Diethyl phthalate is not part of the chain of chemicals that compose the plastic, so it doesn't bind tightly, which means it can be released easily into its surroundings. Surprisingly, diethyl phthalate is also used in a number of personal care products, including skin care, hairspray, nail polish, deodorant, and perfume. It is used to make smells and colors last longer, but it's a known EDC.

You can find this information in the CDC's Agency for Toxic Substances and Disease Registry (ATSDR). Liver tumors were seen in mice after DEP was placed directly on their skin daily for two years. Animal studies have also linked exposure to this chemical with liver and kidney impairment, birth defects, skin sensitivity, and offspring born with an extra rib. These studies haven't been done in humans, but I surely wouldn't want to be part of that study—would you?

Despite what research suggests, these chemicals have penetrated many people's skin. A March 2014 study published in the

> *"Fragrances can contain a number of endocrine disrupting chemicals (EDCs) and are among the top five allergens in the world."*

journal *Environmental Health Perspectives* found metabolites of diethyl phthalate and other phthalates in more than 75 percent of the samples from the National Health and Nutrition Examination Survey (NHANES). That number suggests widespread exposure and absorption of phthalates in the United States. Canadians aren't any better off. A November 2013 study published in the *International Journal of Hygiene and International Health* noted that eleven phthalate metabolites were detected in more than 90 percent of Canadians surveyed in the Canadian Health Measures Survey 2007 to 2009.

Some experts argue we need more research on phthalates and human health, but what we already know may be shocking enough to make you think twice about what you use on your skin. For example, the NHANES suggested a correlation between high phthalate metabolite levels and abdominal obesity and insulin resistance among the study group. Phthalates have also been linked to a number of health problems, such as obesity, autism, puberty changes, and infertility.

Fragrance is everywhere in personal care products, but you can still smell great without the toxicity concerns of synthetic fragrances.

#2 INGREDIENT TO AVOID: FORMALDEHYDE RELEASERS

Look for formaldehyde releasers on skin care labels: quaternium-15, diazolidinyl urea, DMDM hydantoin, bronopol, or imidazolidinyl urea. These ingredients are called formaldehyde releasers because they release formaldehyde into the surrounding air and liquids. In other words, when you rub skin care products containing these chemicals onto your skin, they can be released into the air you breathe, or penetrate your skin and enter your system.

Formaldehyde is known to cause DNA damage and cancer. It is most dangerous when inhaled and, in liquid form, can be absorbed through the skin. In addition to being carcinogenic, formaldehyde and its releasers can cause "allergic" reactions, including skin irritations and asthma.

The FDA has provided data noting that close to one-fifth of all cosmetics in the United States contain formaldehyde releasers, and an April 2010 study published in the journal *Contact Dermatitis* suggests that number may be higher.

While some say exposure to a small amount of this ingredient is "safe," I'm skeptical. We're exposed to formaldehyde through common pressed-wood furniture, building materials, permanent-press fabrics, paper product coatings, glues and adhesives, cigarette smoke, and vehicle exhaust. We're already surrounded by this component—and the American Cancer Society has pointed out high levels of exposure may be carcinogenic to humans—so *why increase that exposure when we don't have to?* In skin care products, formaldehyde releasers are used as preservatives, but the good news is there are natural alternatives!

#3 INGREDIENT TO AVOID: MINERAL OIL

Both untreated and mildly treated mineral oils are in this category. Look for these on skin care labels: mineral oil, liquid petroleum, paraffin oil, and white mineral oil. Mineral oil is derived from crude oil and is in a variety of skin care products and cosmetics. In addition to being a nonrenewable source and not environmentally friendly, some research suggests concerns about its safety. The Campaign for Safe Cosmetics has classified untreated and mildly treated mineral oils as known human carcinogens. They contain harmful impurities, such as polyaromatic hydrocarbons (PAHs), which are carcinogenic. Cosmetic-grade mineral oil is supposed to be purified and free of these carcinogens, but research suggests it may not be as safe as claimed.

While most mineral oils in personal care products are refined and considered "safe," they're still derived from crude oil, so I'm not convinced we should be slathering them on our bodies. They do accumulate in our bodies. An October 2014 study in the journal *Food and Chemical Toxicology* suggests they reach our fat, lymph nodes, liver, spleen, and lungs. And that accumulation appears to be from skin care products such as sunscreen, lipstick, and hand cream. "There is strong evidence that mineral oil hydrocarbons are the greatest contaminant of the human body, amounting to approximately 1 gram per person," write the authors of a November 2011 study published in the *Journal of Women's Health*. That study evaluated 142 pregnant women, testing fat and milk samples for mineral oil–saturated hydrocarbons (MOSH). Study participants completed a questionnaire on their use of cosmetics, and researchers drew a link between hydrocarbon accumulation and use of these products.

Lipsticks and lip-care products may be a particular source of exposure. An April 2016 study published in the *International Journal of Cosmetic Science* found 175 cosmetic lip products contained MOSH and +POSH (polyolefin oligomeric saturated hydrocarbons), and their levels exceeded the recommendations of Cosmetics Europe.

Mineral oil is an inexpensive lubricant for manufacturers, but there are no clear benefits for skin. There are much healthier, natural, eco-friendly, and effective alternatives I'll share with you.

#4 INGREDIENT TO AVOID: PARABENS

To identify parabens on skin care labels, look for propylparaben, benzylparaben, methylparaben, or butylparaben.

Parabens are known xenoestrogens, which means they have estrogenic activity in the body. A 2004 study published in the *Journal of Applied Toxicology* detected parabens in breast tumors and discussed the estrogen-like properties of parabens. Parabens have been found in breast tumors, yet many skin care companies deny this means anything for consumers' health. While this study does not necessarily show that parabens directly cause breast cancer, we do know from this research that parabens are absorbed through the skin and can be taken up and stored in our body tissues, including the breasts.

A study published in *Environmental Health Perspectives* concluded, "Parabens might be active at exposure levels not previously considered toxicologically relevant from studies testing their effects in isolation." This

> *"Parabens have been found in breast tumors, yet many skin care companies deny this means anything for consumers' health."*

suggests parabens are not as benign as some manufacturers claim.

We know parabens are absorbed from our skin care products. The EWG did a study of teenage girls, and *all* participants tested positive for two parabens: methylparaben and propylparaben. I have seen the same thing in my professional experience. I looked at levels of ten women using popular skin care products daily and found 100 percent had detectable levels of parabens in their urine. For most of them, I noticed clear connections between their urine levels and the exact paraben type in the skin care products they were using. When they changed their skin care to The Spa Dr.'s Daily Essentials, I saw a shift in all of those detectable levels. It's time for skin care companies to stop denying the concerns about parabens, and, as consumers, it's our job to read labels and demand change.

#5 INGREDIENT TO AVOID: DEA (DIETHA-NOLAMINE), MEA (MONOETHANOLAMIDE), AND TEA (TRIETHANOLAMINE)

DEA, MEA, and TEA will appear on your skin care labels just this way. These ingredients are used to make skin care products such as moisturizers and sunscreens creamy, and cleansers and soaps foamy, and help increase the pH of the formula. But these are unnecessary because there are safe, natural alternatives.

Studies have shown a link between exposure to high doses of these chemicals and liver cancers, and precancerous changes in skin and the thyroid. Canada and the European Union classify DEA, for example, as harmful and toxic. But it's still used regularly in the United States.

These ingredients can also react with other chemicals in cosmetics to form carcinogenic nitrosamines. So if you're not convinced they're toxic on their own, data suggests that when combined with other common skin care ingredients, the resulting chemical reaction makes them carcinogenic.

*

Unfortunately, these five ingredients are just a start! There are many more ingredients in skin care products that are toxic and harmful to your health. I've compiled a longer list of twenty ingredients, and there are still others—some we know about and others that are only now emerging. Some research has revealed the toxicity of certain skin care ingredients, but more needs to be done.

NATURAL ALTERNATIVES

At this point, you may think there's no escaping potential harm. The good news is there are healthier alternatives, which I'm about to share with you. Despite what naysayers claim, natural preservatives, thickeners, and fragrances can provide the results you want without risking your internal and external well-being. I've seen what natural skin care can do for my patients, and their testimonials are what led me to create my own skin care line, The Spa Dr.'s Daily Essentials skin care system—which is clean, nontoxic, and effective, and has a two-year shelf life.

These are the top twenty harmful ingredients (there are many more) to look for in your personal care products. If your products contain these, I suggest throwing them out. Remember, the EU has banned more than 1,000 ingredients for a reason. For more information on these and other ingredients in personal care products, visit the Campaign for Safe Cosmetics website: SafeCosmetics.org.

1. Fragrance: Avoid all fragrance unless it's natural, such as from pure essential oils.

2. Formaldehyde and formaldehyde releasers (quaternium-15, diazolidinyl urea, DMDM hydantoin, bronopol, or imidazolidinyl urea): A known carcinogen and irritant found in nail products, hair dye, hair straighteners, false eyelash adhesives, and some shampoos.

3. Mineral oil and petroleum (also called petrolatum, petroleum jelly, and paraffin oil): Made from petroleum; research suggests contamination with this ingredient may be linked with cancer.

4. Parabens (propyl-, isopropyl-, butyl-, and isobutyl-): Used in many personal care products as preservatives, parabens have been found in breast tumor tissue and have estrogenic activity.

5. Ethanolamines (diethanolamine [DEA], monoethanolamine [MEA], and triethanolamine [TEA]): Studies link these with cancer, especially when combined with other ingredients that form nitrosamines.

6. Oxybenzone (benzophenone), octinoxate, and homosalate: Found in many sunscreens, lip balms, and other products with SPF, these chemicals may have hormone-disrupting effects. In 2008 the CDC reported that oxybenzone was found in the urine of 97 percent of people tested, so we know it's easily absorbed. Studies also show oxybenzone can build up in fatty tissues and is linked to allergic reactions.

7. Hydroquinone (or tocopheryl acetate) and other skin lighteners: The FDA warns that hydroquinone can cause a skin disease called ochronosis with "disfiguring and irreversible" blue-black lesions on exposed skin. In addition, hydroquinone has been linked to an increased risk of skin cancer. These are found in certain cleansers, moisturizers, and other "skin-lightening" products. Illegally imported skin lighteners can also contain mercury.

(continued)

8. Butylated hydroxyanisole (BHA): Used as a preservative and stabilizer in personal care products. The U.S. National Toxicology Program, a part of the National Institutes of Health, has classified BHA as "reasonably anticipated to be a human carcinogen" based upon outcomes in animal studies. It has also been labeled as a hormone disruptor.

9. Triclosan and triclocarban: Used as antimicrobial agents in personal care products, such as soaps. The CDC found them in the urine of 75 percent of people tested, due to widespread use of antimicrobial cleaning products. Triclosan has been linked to hormone disruption, development of antibacterial resistance, and environmental concerns. The American Medical Association and the American Academy of Microbiology say soap and water serve just as well to prevent the spread of infections and reduce bacteria on the skin.

10. Coal tar ingredients (including aminophenol, diaminobenzene, and phenylenediamine): Used in creams, ointments, soaps, and shampoos to address itchy, scaly skin. These ingredients are derived from tar, a known human carcinogen, according to the National Toxicology Program and the International Agency for Research on Cancer.

11. Toluene: This volatile petrochemical solvent and paint thinner is also used in nail products. It is neurotoxic and an irritant that can impair breathing and cause nausea. Human epidemiological studies and animal studies have linked this ingredient with toxicity to the immune system and certain cancers.

12. Mica, silica (crystalline), talc (unless asbestos free), and nanoparticled titanium dioxide (TiO_2) in powders, loose makeups, or spray: These ingredients may be risky when used in powders or sprays because their tiny particle sizes are easily inhaled and can lodge inside our bodies and irritate our lungs. Over time, this effect may lead to lung disease. Note that these ingredients do not have the same potential harms when used in creams and lotions—in other words, when they aren't inhaled.

13. Methylisothiazolinone, methylchloroisothiazolinone, and benzisothiazolinone (also 2-methyl-4-isothiazoline-3-one, Neolone 950 preservative, MI, OriStar MIT, and Microcare MT, 5-Chloro-2-methyl-4-isothiazolin-3-one and MCI): Commonly used as chemical preservatives in personal care products, they may pose a risk for organ toxicity and allergic reactions.

14. Heavy metals, such as mercury, lead, arsenic, and aluminum: May be added to products, but most often they're present due to contamination of ingredients from the environment. Therefore, heavy metals may not be on the ingredient label. Look for calomel, lead acetate, mercurio, mercuri chloride, or thimerosal. With accumulations in the body over time, heavy metals can impair the brain and nervous system, disrupt hormones, and potentially cause cancer.

15. Resorcinol (or 1,3-benzenediol, resorcin, 1,3-dihydroxybenzene, m-hydroxybenze, m-dihydroxyphenol): Used in tire production and a common ingredient in hair color, bleaching, and certain acne and eczema peels and treatments. It is a known skin irritant and allergen. Some research also suggests it's toxic to the immune system, and animal studies have linked exposure to this ingredient with thyroid disruption.

16. Carbon black (or D & C Black No. 2, channel black, acetylene black, furnace black, lamp black, and thermal black): Used as a pigment in certain makeup and nail polish, it has been linked to cancer and toxicity for certain organs, including the skin.

17. P-phenylenediamine (or 4-aminoaniline; 1,4-benzenediamine; p-diamino-benzene; 1,4-diaminobenzene; 1,4-phenylene diamine): These are plastics used in hair dyes. Research suggests they can cause skin reactions, organ system toxicity, and possibly cancer.

18. Teflon (and polytetrafluoroethylene [PTFE], polyperfluoromethyliso-propyl ether, DEA-C8-18 perfluoroalkylethyl phosphate): The same substance that commonly coats nonstick cookware, it's sometimes used in makeup. Teflon may be contaminated with PFOAs, which have been associated with cancer and hormone disruption. Stay away from these ingredients in cookware as well as cosmetics.

19. Acrylamide (also polyacrylamide; polyacrylate, polyquaternium, acry-late): Used in certain creams, lotions, makeup, sunscreen, and hair care products as a stabilizing and binding agent. Acrylamide is a potential human carcinogen and has been shown to disrupt reproduction in animal studies.

20. Phenoxyethanol (also Euxyl K® 400 and PhE): This chemical preservative is used in a variety of personal care products, such as perfume, makeups, hand sanitiz-ers, deodorants, toothpaste, baby wipes, sunscreens, and lotions. It has been linked to skin irritation, eczema, and even central nervous system effects.

USING ESSENTIAL OILS SAFELY

Essential oils are powerful and healing when used properly. There are a few things to keep in mind to obtain the maximum benefits and avoid any potential harm.

- **Check for purity.** Only use essential oils with the absolute highest standards. The oil should not feel greasy, smell like alcohol, or smell rancid. Some essential oils are extracted with harmful practices. Ask questions about the purity and concentration. Be wary of low-priced essential oils. Look for those labeled organic or wild crafted.

- **Do a patch test.** Some people are sensitive to essential oils and may develop contact dermatitis or skin irritation. If your skin is sensitive, apply the product to a small area of your inner forearm and place an adhesive bandage over it. If you develop a rash, redness, or itchiness within twenty-four hours, you may have a sensitivity and should reconsider using the product.

- **Start small and simple.** Generally it's best to start with 2 to 3 drops per application. I use a carrier oil, such as coconut, almond, or jojoba oil, and mix 1 or 2 drops of the essential oil in 2 to 5 tablespoons (30 to 75 ml) of the carrier oil. I don't recommend applying essential oils straight (without diluting) at first. Some oils are stronger than others; dilute those even more.

- **Use caution in the sun when using citrus essential oils.** Furanocoumarin, a chemical component in citrus peel, is responsible for sun sensitivity (e.g., easy burning or excess pigmentation). There is risk of potentially serious damage when it's on skin exposed to sunlight. If you're using skin care products with citrus essential oils, make sure they're furanocoumarin free.

- **Use caution when using straight (undiluted) essential oils.** This is particularly important if you are pregnant, nursing, or want to use essential oils on your child. Certain components of essential oils, such as ketones, can be great for healing but can be neurotoxic to sensitive patients, such as people with seizure disorders, pregnant women, and babies.

- **Work with a specialist.** If you have specific health or skin issues, it's best to work with a qualified health care provider to ensure you get the best care possible and your condition is safely monitored. If you want to use essential oils therapeutically, consider working with someone who is well trained in their use.

ESSENTIAL OILS FOR SKIN

Essential oils have long been known for their therapeutic effects and powerful natural fragrance. There are numerous fantastic essential oils for skin and overall health. I'll share my six favorites. Of course there are many more essential oils with therapeutic and naturally fragrant properties. Peppermint, lemon balm, lemongrass, jasmine, and frankincense essential oils all have skin-enhancing and healing benefits too. I could go on, but the following six essential oils offer a good starting point for incorporating them into your everyday skin care as fragrance alternatives or for their therapeutic benefits.

TEA TREE OIL ESSENTIAL OIL

While perhaps not a favorite scent, tea tree oil has antimicrobial and anti-inflammatory properties, and it is well known to help reduce breakouts in patients with mild to moderate acne. In addition to helping acne, research shows tea tree oil can be effective for addressing seborrheic dermatitis and chronic gingivitis (gum disease), as well as speeding the wound-healing process. Because of its antifungal and antiviral effects, tea tree oil may also help with warts and fungal infections such as athlete's foot and nail fungus. It has also been shown to have antibacterial activity against the bacterium MRSA.

YLANG-YLANG FLOWER ESSENTIAL OIL

This essential oil has a beautifully exotic, sweet smell and a euphoric, sedative effect on the nervous system. It often helps relieve tension and stress. Topically, ylang-ylang oil helps with sebum balance for both overly dry and overly oily complexions. It has an amazing ability to help maintain proper moisture levels by preventing skin's water loss, which in turn makes skin appear resilient and smooth. It also has a soothing effect. It is one of the star oils in The Spa Dr.'s Daily Essentials proprietary 100 percent organic, natural essential oil blend.

BERGAMOT FRUIT ESSENTIAL OIL

This oil has a lovely natural fragrance, as well as antiseptic and antibacterial properties. It can help regulate sebum secretion and is known to help even skin tone and promote wound healing. Blemishes of all types can benefit with topical application of this oil. Because this is a citrus oil, it's important to be careful about sun exposure after usage. You can apply it in the evenings in small amounts, but some people continue to have sun sensitivity effects twenty-four hours after use. The Spa Dr.'s skin care uses only furocoumarin-free or bergapten-free bergamot oil.

MAY CHANG PEEL ESSENTIAL OIL

This oil is widely used in traditional Chinese medicine for its anti-congestive, antiseptic, and calming benefits. In today's skin care, this oil helps address oily skin and breakouts thanks to its astringent, antimicrobial, and anti-inflammatory action. May Chang peel oil is known for its deeply cleansing and pore-reducing effects without irritating or drying skin. It's soothing and healing, and its amazing smell makes it the perfect natural fragrance, which is why we also include this in The Spa Dr.'s Daily Essentials proprietary 100 percent organic, natural fragrance.

CLARY SAGE ESSENTIAL OIL

Clary sage oil contains natural antimicrobial agents, so it can be helpful with wounds and skin infections. Research published in February 2015 in the journal *Postępy Dermatologii i Alergologii* showed it can help fight certain staphylococcus-caused skin infections. While these types of skin infections are common, see your doctor if your infection is serious or continues for more than a few days without signs of improvement.

LAVENDER ESSENTIAL OIL

This popular essential oil is known for its stress-reducing, soothing, and calming properties, as well as its antimicrobial capabilities against bacteria, fungi, and yeasts. Research shows it also has anti-inflammatory and immune-boosting effects. These benefits, plus pain-reducing and wound-healing properties, make lavender one of my favorite remedies in skin care.

NATURAL PRESERVATIVES

Natural preservatives, such as citric acid, gluconolactone, and rosemary leaf extract, work great as part of a healthier preservative system in natural skin care products. We need preservatives to prevent products from growing mold, the wrong bacteria, and other harmful microorganisms. If we use products containing contaminants, it may disrupt our skin microbiome and can lead to breakouts and infections, some of which can be quite serious.

In chapter 9, you will find DIY skin care recipes, which do not contain preservatives. Because of that, you will need to make a fresh batch every few days. If you want something a little more long-term and convenient, I will cover premade natural skin care products in chapter 10.

Some natural preservatives we use in The Spa Dr.'s Daily Essentials include:

▸ **ROSEMARY LEAF EXTRACT:** High antioxidant, anti-inflammatory, and antimicrobial properties work beautifully as part of a natural preservative system. Instead of harming our skin and health, it actually helps make our skin smooth and soft.

▸ **CITRIC ACID:** Naturally found in lemons and limes, it helps prevent bacterial overgrowth. When used at very low levels, and when carefully prepared, it can also help regulate acidity of skin care products to match the skin's natural pH. Too much citric acid can make the pH of products too low and cause sun sensitivity, so manufacturing practices are important.

▸ **GLUCONOLACTONE:** Derived and produced by the oxidation of glucose by microorganisms, it has broad-spectrum protection that improves skin moisture, an exceptional low-toxicity profile, and a long history of use. Plus, it is nonsensitizing and nonirritating.

NONTOXIC OILS

Many of the base oils in popular skin care products—such as mineral oil—are used because they're inexpensive and have a long shelf life. However, as already noted, mineral oil comes from petroleum and poses safety risks.

In the past, people typically steered away from applying oils to skin due to the belief they clogged pores and caused breakouts. We now know not all oils are bad. Just like there are good fats for our inner nourishment, there are good oils to use externally for our skin health.

SIX FAVORITE NONTOXIC CARRIER OILS FOR DIY TOPICAL SKIN CARE

Remember, not all oils are the same, so choose the right ones. Also, use only extra-virgin cold-pressed oils, and ensure they are clean, pure, and not rancid.

1. Coconut oil is one of nature's best moisturizers and emollients thanks to its medium-chain triglycerides that keep skin smooth, protected, and hydrated. It works well to remove makeup and surface buildup.

Coconut oil is rich in capric, caprylic, and lauric fatty acids, which have strong disinfectant and antimicrobial properties. Some people with acne-prone skin believe they're not able to use coconut oil, but I find it depends on the quality of the coconut oil and the other ingredients you combine it with. The key when using coconut oil on any skin type is to use a pure, extra-virgin source. Unlike other oils, coconut oil does not easily become rancid, so it stays fresh longer.

2. Sunflower seed oil is a light-colored oil that comes from the seeds of the sunflower plant. The oil provides a rich source of unsaturated linoleic and oleic fatty acids, plus vitamin E. Sunflower seed oil is soothing and calming to skin. It is thinner than some other oils, so it works well in combination to make other oils easier to apply.

3. Sweet almond oil is pressed from the nut kernels of the sweet almond tree. This light and mildly scented oil is gentle on skin and easily absorbed. Due to its high content of essential fatty acids, it protects from drying and improves the skin's barrier function, keeping it smooth and supple. This is a great oil to use for blending in DIY recipes.

4. Avocado oil has been used for centuries for beauty and skin care. Rich in vitamins A and E and highly absorptive, this oil is great for dry or mature skin. In addition to its hydrating qualities, its high antioxidant levels help heal and protect skin. I prefer extra-virgin over the refined avocado oil found in the cooking oil section of your grocery store. The extra-virgin oil has a green hue, which indicates its naturally occurring chlorophyll—an added benefit for skin!

5. Apricot kernel oil is rich in vitamins A, C, and E, plus various minerals, as well as omega-6 and -9 fatty acids. Its lightweight consistency absorbs fast without leaving a greasy residue. Suitable for even the most sensitive skin types, including babies, its soothing and anti-inflammatory properties provide relief for such conditions as acne, eczema, and dermatitis. It is an excellent repairing, revitalizing, nourishing, and softening agent that restores skin's smoothness and suppleness.

6. Argan kernel oil is extracted from the kernels of the Moroccan argan tree and is rich in vitamin E, fatty acids (vitamin F), carotenoids such as beta-carotene, and phytosterols. Thanks to its antioxidant content, it can ward off aging signs in our skin. It supports skin's natural mild acidity, imparts softness, and protects against dryness. Argan oil is a noncomedogenic, anti-inflammatory, and regenerative agent, so it can also be used with oily and acne-prone skin types. It is often recommended for various skin irritations, scars, stretch marks, and sunburns. Argan oil is also known to protect and heal dry, brittle hair and nails.

In chapter 9, we'll talk more about creating your own blend of these natural ingredients to suit your needs and preferences. Again, I emphasize it's essential to *use organic, extra-virgin cold-pressed forms* to obtain the cleanest oils with all the best nutrients. Processed and refined oils have been stripped of most (or all) of their healing properties.

You will find most of these oils in The Spa Dr.'s Daily Essentials. To help ensure the oils remain fresh, we add a mix of tocopherols (vitamin E). Our tocopherols are made from GMO-free sunflower seed oil and provide antioxidant protection to oils. Vitamin E itself is a potent antioxidant and an excellent skin protectant.

PLANT-BASED SKIN SOOTHERS

Instead of potentially toxic ingredients, such as coal tar for dry, scaly, irritated skin, you can choose natural skin soothers, such as aloe and arnica. In chapter 3, I covered two of my favorite natural skin care ingredients: pineapple (*Ananas sativus*) fruit extract (see page 37), and green algae (*Chlorella vulgaris*) extract (see page 37). Here are a few more favorites:

ALOE VERA LEAF

Aloe vera has the ability to effectively penetrate and transport healthy substances through the skin. Aloe vera provides numerous cutaneous skin benefits, such as being an excellent moisturizer, keeping skin flexible, and supplying oxygen to cells. It also increases the strength and synthesis of skin tissue, preventing premature aging. Rich in mucopolysaccharides (naturally occurring sugars that keep skin moist and plump), minerals, amino acids, and enzymes, aloe has renowned soothing, anti-inflammatory, and healing properties, making it a great option for treating cuts, grazes, insect bites, sunburn, acne, dermatitis, and sensitive and irritated skin.

BLACK TEA LEAF

Black tea leaf has about double the caffeine content of green tea, which can help reduce skin's redness and puffiness, as well as protect it against sun damage. Black tea extract is a good-quality antibacterial astringent; regular application can help control breakouts of pimples and even acne.

WHITE AND GREEN TEA LEAVES

Both white and green tea leaves come from the same plant, so it's only natural they share some benefits. White tea is produced from the youngest tea leaves and is minimally processed. Both types encourage longer moisture retention for your skin. Combine that with potent antiaging compounds, and they're an excellent resource for keeping fine lines and wrinkles at bay. They can also help brighten and even your complexion because of their cleansing effects, and their naturally occurring catechins have anti-inflammatory properties. Parabens deactivate green tea polyphenols—another reason to avoid them.

TURMERIC (*Curcuma longa*) ROOT

Turmeric is a South Indian spice with a long-standing use as a flavoring and coloring agent, as well as a medicinal and beautifying herb. Turmeric has scientifically proven anti-inflammatory and soothing properties that help relieve inflammation, redness, and itchiness. Turmeric manages microorganism growth on the skin, helping ward off acne-causing *P. acnes* bacteria and prevents other infections from spreading. It also contains powerful antioxidant properties, balances sebum secretion, and helps clean out pores. Turmeric has been clinically shown to control the psoriasis causing T-lymphocyte autoimmune proliferation.

SIBERIAN GINSENG (*Eleutherococcus senticosus*) ROOT

Ginseng is a powerful adaptogenic medicinal plant that can help increase overall resistance to all types of stress and help rejuvenate and invigorate tired-looking skin.

FIVE NATURAL INGREDIENTS FOR YOUR SKIN FROM YOUR KITCHEN

Here are five of my favorite ingredients you can find in your kitchen that will nourish your skin on the outside without exposing your body to any harmful chemicals (barring any food allergies unique to your skin). You'll find these ingredients and many more in the DIY recipes included in chapter 9.

AVOCADO

Avocado is packed with hydrating oils and skin-nourishing vitamins A and E. If you can resist eating it, a ripe avocado can be instantly transformed into a moisturizing mask. It is one of my favorite ingredients for DIY face masks because it is high in antioxidants and has moisturizing and penetrating benefits.

Allergy alert: If you have an avocado allergy, do not apply it to your face. If you have an allergy to latex, you may also be sensitive to avocados, bananas, green papayas, and kiwi, so start with a skin patch test on your arm before applying it to your face.

NATURAL HONEY

Honey, a natural humectant, helps retain moisture and regulate pH, making it a perfect ingredient in skin care. In addition to honey's cosmetic benefits, it has powerful antimicrobial and anti-inflammatory properties, meaning it's helpful for wound healing and a number of skin conditions. In fact, according to a December 2013 study published in the *Journal of Cosmetic Dermatology*, historical records show honey has been used for healing and cosmetics since the earliest civilizations (even as far back as 4500 BCE in Egypt).

Honey has many healing benefits and is rich in amino acids, enzymes, biotin, vitamins B_1, B_3, B_5, and B_6, potassium, and calcium. In food and skin care, use raw (unpasteurized) honey, as you don't want to kill the beneficial bacteria or remove the nutrients. Darker honeys tend to have higher antioxidant levels. Acacia and Manuka honey seem to have the most therapeutic effects, but any raw honey can be used, especially if you have a local source.

OATS

Oats provide moisturizing, healing, and anti-inflammatory skin benefits. Due to their saponin content, oats work well to cleanse skin without drying it out. In addition, their antioxidant and hydrating qualities make them a great addition to face masks. Because oats have skin-soothing and itch-reducing properties, they also help soothe inflamed, irritated skin and heal eczema and hives.

YOGURT

Yogurt contains nutrients, enzymes, and active cultures that can aid in smoothing and balancing your skin. Lactic acid (an alpha-hydroxyl acid) helps dissolve dead skin cells for natural exfoliation to help smooth and rejuvenate. The natural acidity of yogurt also balances skin's mildly acidic pH, and its beneficial microorganisms may help support your skin's microbiome. Yogurt's properties also have the ability to sooth irritated and inflamed skin. Topically, you can choose any type of yogurt—cow's milk, sheep's milk, goat's milk, coconut milk, or other variety—as long as it is unsweetened and plain.

PAPAYA

Papaya is rich in vitamins A, C, and E, which are nourishing and protective. Papaya's natural enzyme papain helps exfoliate skin, leaving it smooth and soft. These are the reasons

> *"Nature provides us with natural actives that have powerful abilities to help clear, rejuvenate, and heal skin."*

papaya is one of my favorite DIY skin care ingredients. Not only does it naturally exfoliate your skin, but it also hydrates and can reduce signs of aging, such as fine lines, wrinkles, and hyperpigmentation. Greener, less-ripe papayas have higher amounts of papain. For sensitive skin types, I suggest using ripe papayas because they're less likely to trigger an inflammatory reaction.

As you can see, nature provides us with natural actives that have powerful abilities to help clear, rejuvenate, and heal skin. In addition to avoiding harmful effects of potentially toxic chemicals in common skin care products, choosing natural solutions enhances your skin's appearance and your natural beauty.

YOUR DAILY RITUAL

Creating a daily ritual helps awaken skin in the morning and restore skin while you're sleeping. I recommend these three steps in your daily routine:

1. Cleanse in the morning to remove perspiration and balance oils and microorganisms on your skin. At night, a cleanser should remove any makeup and debris (sweat, dirt, and pollution residue) from the day. While it should effectively clean, it should NOT strip

your skip of its beneficial oils, microbiome, or damage the delicate pH balance.

2. Nourish with a toner or serum. Toners can help rebalance skin pH after water and cleansers have touched your face. If you have a mildly acidic pH cleanser, you may not need a toner for this purpose. A well-made toner or serum can saturate skin with antioxidants and other nutrients to help nourish and protect it. Apply this in the morning to revitalize skin and prepare for the day, and again at night to rebalance your skin.

3. Moisturize both morning and night to hydrate and plump skin with natural actives. Many moisturizers simply sit on the surface and make you look glowy while you're wearing them but do not have a lasting effect. You may use heavy or light moisturizers, depending on your preference and skin type. My skin care system offers one moisturizer for all skin types, as well as a fourth step I call "glow boost" because it contains a blend of organic extra-virgin cold-pressed oils that provide extra hydration and antioxidant benefit for a natural glow.

In the morning, you should also add a sunblock. Avoid hormone-disrupting chemicals such as oxybenzone, and opt instead for a mineral-based makeup and/or sunblock containing zinc oxide.

Exfoliation is another important part of the skin care routine, but not as a daily practice. Gentle exfoliation once a week can help slough off dead skin and enhance the effectiveness of your daily three steps.

Now that you know how to achieve a clean slate, let's move on to the rest of your body and your mind.

CHAPTER 5

Clean Body and Clean Mind

Now, with a clean plate and a clean slate, it's time to focus on achieving a clean body and clean mind. A clean body comes from reducing additional triggers in your surroundings that can inflame and irritate skin, as well as enhancing your body's detoxification pathways to clean and clear skin from the inside out.

Along the same lines, because stress is toxic, we can develop a clean mind by reducing emotional upset and worry, balancing hormones, and aligning with our highest purpose so our inner beauty shines through. A clean plate, slate, body, and mind, ultimately, are what lead to clean skin, graceful aging, natural beauty, and the confidence that come with them.

CLEAN BODY

As you're now aware, we are regularly exposed to toxins in our air, water, food, and personal care products. Food additives, plasticizers, chemical solvents, heavy metal–based pesticides, herbicides, and pharmaceutical drugs possess endocrine-disrupting effects that can lead to chronic skin and health problems, so it's important to reduce our overall exposure as much as possible.

REDUCING TOXINS IN YOUR HOME AND FOOD

The first step to achieving a clean body is to reduce your exposure to other environmental toxins in your home and food. I know that task may sound daunting, but don't worry. I'll share some easy ways to eliminate exposures to toxins in air, water, and food. Focus on your home and the food you eat, because these are the areas you have the most control over.

EIGHT WAYS TO REDUCE TOXINS IN YOUR HOME

Our homes are our havens, and we'd hate to think they contribute any danger to our well-being. Follow these simple tips to keep them toxin-free.

1. Remove your shoes when entering your home. Walking around outside, we pick up all sorts of chemicals and germs on our shoes. At the park, we may pick up pesticides and dog feces, and you may step through gasoline residue at the gas station.

You may then bring these toxins into your home on your shoes—unless you leave them at the door.

2. Change your central-air filters once a month, and have the air ducts cleaned. Consistently changing the air filters and having the ducts cleaned can help improve your home's air quality. Changing air filters once a month is a good rule of thumb; you may be able to get away with cleaning air ducts once a year, but it depends on how often you use your central air-conditioning. If you have allergies, live in a major city, or live in a closed-up home during cold winter months, consider putting high-quality air filters in your bedroom or living room. To go above and beyond, do both. Using a combination high-efficiency particulate arresting (HEPA) and ionizing air filter can further reduce allergens and pollutants in your air. Austin, IQ Air, and Blue Air are some of my favorite combination filtration units.

3. Reduce moisture to avoid mold growth. Moisture lurking in walls and floors from water damage or leaks can lead to the growth of toxic mold over time. Mold growth in homes is more common than you may realize and can trigger a number of health issues, including chronic skin problems. Check your home for plumbing leaks, and keep irrigation at least two feet from the exterior walls of your home. If you notice damage, have it repaired as soon as possible. If you suspect mold, or have a history of water damage in your home, contact an environmental specialist for mold testing.

4. Use nontoxic cleaning products. Most popular cleaning products are full of harmful chemicals that can release into the air and leave behind toxic residues. You and your family may inhale and touch these chemicals for days afterward. Look for healthier, more environmentally friendly alternatives at your local health food store or online. Or consider this frugal home-made option: Baking soda, lemon juice, and vinegar will clean just about everything in your house.

5. Do not let your car idle in an attached garage. The car exhaust can seep around the door to your home and become trapped inside. This effect is enhanced on a cold day, when the temperature difference pulls the cold air from your garage (and its smells) into your warm home. After you start your car, back out of the garage without idling. As a bonus, it's best for the environment to avoid idling whenever possible.

6. Be wary of what you bring into your home. Furniture, carpeting, rugs, and building materials can be full of chemicals that release toxins into your home and contribute to indoor air pollution. When purchasing items for your home, look for natural materials or options made with "green" construction.

7. Wash new clothes before wearing them. The majority of clothing manufactured today is treated with numerous chemicals, such as antiwrinkle and fire-retardant chemicals. Some of those chemicals can simply be removed by washing. Along those lines, avoid dry cleaning or switch to a more eco-friendly cleaner to avoid excess exposure to potential toxins.

8. Refrain from using pesticides and other chemicals in your home and yard. Those seemingly harmless bug sprays, insect

repellents, and weed killers contain chemicals that are toxic for humans as well as insects and plants. They linger in the air and your home and can travel inside on your clothes and shoes. Fortunately, multiple natural alternatives are available. For example, make your own weed killer by mixing 1 gallon (3.87 L) of vinegar, 1 cup (288 g) of salt, and 8 drops of liquid soap; then spray it on the weeds.

FIVE WAYS TO REDUCE TOXINS IN YOUR FOOD AND DRINKS

We know what we put into our bodies is reflected on the outside by our skin's health (or woes). So the first step to reducing toxins in foods is to follow my two-week program. Eating a balanced diet with adequate protein and fiber devoid of sugar supports the body's detoxification pathways and elimination of toxins. Avoiding sugar, in particular, is important, as it can make the liver's ability to remove chemicals from the body less efficient. Let's look at what else we can do to keep our food and drinks toxin free.

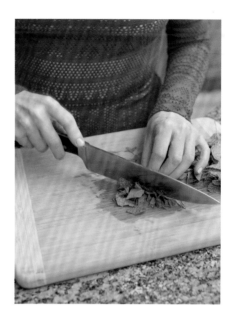

1. Filter your water. Clean water is key for a clean body. If you're not sure what kind of filtration system to get, you can start by having your tap water tested by a local company; if you're on a public water supply, check your area's water testing through your water company. Carbon filters can help reduce some chemicals, such as chlorine, fluorine, and pesticides. My favorite for drinking water is Reverse Osmosis, which removes these and other microorganisms and chemicals for pure water. Also consider a whole-house filtration system or shower and bath filter to reduce topical exposure to chlorine and other chemicals that can affect your skin and overall health.

2. Use glass, ceramic, or stainless steel containers for storage. Food and drinks stored in plastic may become contaminated with leached chemicals, such as BPA and phthalates. Reduce your exposure to these hormone-disrupting chemicals by storing your food and beverages in glass, ceramic, or stainless steel.

3. Use stainless steel, glass, ceramic, or cast iron for cooking. Avoid Teflon or other "nonstick" cookware with perfluorooctanoic acid (PFOA) and other chemicals linked to cancer and other health concerns.

4. Choose organic as much as possible. Certain crops are heavily sprayed or hold onto pesticides more than other produce. Peeling may help, but some skins are thin and still end up in the parts you consume. Ideally,

we'd always choose organic, local produce, but these tend to be more expensive than regular produce. But if you're on a budget and can't always afford organic produce, ewg.org has a "dirty dozen" and "clean fifteen" list of fruits and veggies that can help you determine which produce to prioritize when buying organic.

5. Choose animal products from sustainably and naturally raised animals. Meats, fish, and other animal protein that are free range, grass fed, and sustainably raised have higher nutritional value than those that aren't. When you choose the organic variety as well, they contain little to no pesticide residue. They're also better for our environment. This includes choosing "cleaner" fish and avoiding large, carnivorous fish higher on the food chain, such as swordfish, shark, tuna, halibut, king mackerel, and tilefish, which contain higher amounts of mercury, PCBs, and other environmental pollutants.

RAMP UP YOUR BODY'S NATURAL DETOXIFICATION PATHWAYS

Once you reduce your exposure to toxins, the next step is ramping up your body's natural detoxification pathways. The most important organs for cleansing are the skin, the lymphatic system, the digestive system, the liver, and the kidneys. The liver is the primary detoxification organ in the body. As it processes about 2 quarts (2 L) of blood every minute, it protects the rest of the body from harmful substances by reducing their toxicity and readying them for excretion.

Our bodies naturally become unbalanced over time due to changes in hormone levels, digestion processes, and differences in nutrition, so it's important to give your detoxification pathways a boost. The two-week program provides a jump-start. Let's discuss how to do this with home spa cleansing techniques.

HOME SPA CLEANSING: FOUR DETOXIFICATION-BOOSTING TECHNIQUES

This is part of the spa cleanse program I have offered at world-renowned spas and have refined over my seventeen years of naturopathic medicine practice. People who do this program have reported clearer, brighter, and youthful-looking skin, as well as weight loss, increased energy, a clearer mind, improved sleep, and reduced pain. While it's wonderful to take time for a spa weekend away, most of us cannot abandon our daily responsibilities for two weeks. That's why I designed this program to do at home—for the everyman and woman—people with busy lives and work schedules to maintain. It includes:

1. Mineral bath

2. Dry skin brushing

3. Castor oil packs/rubs

4. Movement

These four spa-cleansing techniques are easy to do at home, and I'd highly recommend including them in your two-week program. They're designed to enhance detoxification pathways for a clean body, which ultimately helps you achieve clean, glowing skin from within. You can incorporate any or all of these during the two weeks.

MINERAL BATH

Mineral baths have been used for many years to help soothe the body and mind, as well as provide nutrients that support detoxification. You can use bath salts with essential oils or Epsom salts in this relaxing ritual. End your bath with an herbal tea blend that will improve your bath's detox benefits. Dandelion, fennel, milk thistle, burdock root, and yellow dock are some of my favorites for liver and kidney support.

Evenings are a great time to enjoy mineral baths, and you can enjoy these as often as every day during the two-week program. Try to squeeze in at least two or three baths during the plan. If you have irritated skin or a skin condition aggravated by bathing, skip this spa-cleansing technique and see chapter 9 for personalized skin care options, such as the Oatmeal Bath (page 192).

YIELD: 1 bath

Epsom salts or Himalayan salt bath crystals
   (my favorite)
Essential oils of choice, such as lavender, rose,
   or chamomile (optional)
Dried herbs or flowers of choice, such as
   chamomile, elderflower, or rose petals
   (optional)
Herbal tea (optional)

Run a warm bath. Dissolve the salt in the warm water (refer to the packaging for the ratio of salt to water). Add a few drops of essential oil (if using). If you're allergic or sensitive to essential oils, skip this step.

Alternatively, before getting in the tub, place 2 teaspoons (1.3 g) of dried herbs or flowers in 8 ounces (235 ml) of boiling filtered water. Steep for 20 minutes, drain, and then add to your bath.

Enjoy a relaxing soak in the mineral bath (with or without herbs or essential oils) for at least 15 minutes. If you'd like, sip on an herbal tea during your bath to enhance the cleansing process. After bathing, pat skin gently with a towel to dry.

DRY SKIN BRUSHING

Enhance your circulation, improve detoxification, and slough off dead skin with dry skin brushing. Use a long-handled skin brush, available online or at select health food and specialty stores. A great time to do this is before taking a shower. If you have irritated skin, open wounds or eruptions, or severely dry skin, skip this technique or work around affected areas.

YIELD: 1 treatment

While your body is dry, and starting at your toes, brush your skin with your long-handled skin brush in upward strokes toward your heart. Use light to medium pressure. Your skin should tingle but not hurt.

When you reach your belly, start over at your fingers and brush toward your heart, along your arms and up your back. Continue brushing over the entire body (except the head and neck) in movements toward the heart.

Once you've brushed your entire body, take a warm shower and finish with a 5- to 10-second cold shower blast.

CASTOR OIL PACKS/RUBS

Internal use of castor oil is known for its laxative effects, but you can also use it topically for a soothing, cleansing, and nutritive effect. The castor oil pack or rub is placed over the abdomen and liver, whereby the oil is absorbed. It then begins circulating through the lymphatic system.

The castor oil rub is a variation. The best time to do this is at bedtime. You can do this one to four times per week during the two-week program. *Note: Castor oil applications are not recommended during pregnancy and menstruation.*

YIELD: 1 treatment

FOR RUB

Castor oil

FOR PACK

1 flannel pack (available online or at your local health food store)
1 T-shirt or towel you don't mind getting oily and stained
1 hot water bottle

To apply the rub: Apply the castor oil to your hand and then massage it into the area you're treating.

To apply the pack: Saturate the flannel pack with castor oil. Apply the pack to the upper-right quadrant of your abdomen, around the bottom edge of your ribcage near your liver. Alternatively, if you don't have a flannel pack, apply the oil directly. Put on a T-shirt, or cover the application area with a towel.

Lie in bed on your back with your feet elevated. Place pillows under your knees and feet to help relax the abdominal muscles and relieve stress on your lower back. Place the hot water bottle over the affected area. Leave this on for at least 45 minutes to 1 hour. This is an excellent time for visualization, mediation, relaxation exercises, or sleep.

MOVEMENT

Moving your body with exercise is an excellent way to enhance detoxification, but any movement can help increase blood and lymph circulation to enhance cleansing—and, exercise relieves stress! The key is enjoying the exercise you choose as much as possible and doing it every day. Life can get busy, and sometimes it's hard to fit in a yoga class, bike ride, or trip to the gym every day, so choose what fits your schedule. Trust me; your body will thank you for setting aside the time. Yoga is one of my favorites because it's a time-tested technique for strengthening the body and soothing the mind.

If you currently do not exercise regularly or have any physical limitations, check with your doctor to determine which types of exercise are best for you.

YIELD: 1 happy person

10 minutes or more of any of the following activities: running, walking, biking, swimming, fitness classes, yoga, dancing, hula hooping, squats or lunges, jumping jacks, pushups, vacuuming—even yard work

Move your body for at least 10 minutes daily. As your energy and strength improve, increase your exercise intensity and frequency. Your stamina will keep improving to the point where you will be exercising at least 30 minutes every day.

OTHER OPTIONS

If your schedule and budget allow, I recommend seeing practitioners who specialize in acupuncture, acupressure, reflexology, or massage. According to Chinese medicine principles, acupuncture and acupressure (using massage instead of needles) clear blockages in meridians. I find this is a great addition to the two-week program.

Reflexology is another ancient practice that aims to address a number of ailments, including digestive issues and enhancing liver detoxification. The idea behind reflexology is that the bottom of the foot contains reflex points that correspond to the organs of the body.

A full-body massage is also a fantastic option to increase blood and lymph flow to improve your results during the program.

CLEAN MIND

The mind and the skin are closely connected. A number of skin conditions, such as acne, eczema, rosacea, psoriasis, vitiligo, and even premature aging, can both *cause* AND be *triggered by stress*!

Introducing something new into your routine—such as the spa-cleansing techniques—may require you to step outside your comfort zone. These changes can trigger emotional discomfort—so it's important to include supplemental practices for a clean mind. Even if these changes aren't disruptive, a clean mind is an important step in achieving clean skin. It may be tempting to skip the clean mind section because it may seem unrelated to healthy skin, but, as you'll see, it's more closely related than most people realize.

Many of our nerve endings are connected to our skin and other organs. When we experience a heightened sense of emotion, be it sadness, anger, or another upset, these dramatic feelings can play out on our skin. This relationship can be a vicious cycle: Skin problems can affect us on an emotional level, but stress can also affect our skin!

So how does stress affect these different skin conditions? Let's look at the connection in the following conditions.

▸ **Acne:** Stress is not the only cause of acne, but it is a big culprit. When we're stressed, the adrenal glands release the hormone cortisol. A surge in cortisol causes increased sebum production, which triggers acne. Chronically high levels of cortisol can lead to sugar cravings, and eating sugar also increases acne breakouts.

▸ **Eczema:** Anxiety from stress at work, school, and home can make eczema flare. This is partly due to high cortisol levels, which trigger inflammation and aggravate skin inflammation issues, including itchy, irritated skin conditions.

Studies have shown that sleep (or lack of it due to stress) plays a role, affecting our skin's ability to heal eczema. The itching and discomfort eczema causes is stressful and may even keep you awake at night. Unfortunately, those realities only make the problem worse.

▸ **Rosacea:** People with rosacea know that dealing with its visible signs can trigger more flushing, which can lead to more stress. In a National Rosacea Society survey, 70 percent of people with severe rosacea symptoms reported the condition negatively affected their professional interactions, and 41 percent said rosacea compelled them to avoid public contact or cancel social plans.

▸ **Vitiligo:** This autoimmune skin disorder is characterized by white spots or patches. These spots are from lack of pigmentation caused by destruction or weakening of the pigment cells in those areas. Stress is not the direct cause of vitiligo, but it can make the condition worse. We know stress negatively affects our immune system, and being anxious or stressed can aggravate autoimmune conditions (including vitiligo and psoriasis).

▸ **Premature aging:** When we're having a bad day, we usually frown more. While I'm a big fan of smile lines, I don't think anyone likes the look of excessive frown lines, which are likely to occur with chronic stress. High levels of cortisol are likely to cause insomnia, belly fat, and an inability to roll with what life brings our way.

Even if you have seemingly perfect skin, you might not treat it very well when you're under stress. Stressed-out people often develop bad habits, such as picking and rubbing bumps and blemishes, which can lead to permanent scarring. Take a deep breath, and don't stress about these realities!

SIX PRACTICES FOR A CLEAN MIND

During my spiritual psychology training, and over the last seventeen years in clinical practice, I've learned various tools that can help people relieve stress and emotional upset. These are my favorites.

1. Breath work release

2. Forgiveness writing exercise

3. Ten-minute meditation

4. Relaxing bedtime ritual

5. Gratitude journal

6. Nature excursion

Most of these take just ten minutes or less per day—the minimum amount of time I ask of you during the two-week program.

BREATH WORK RELEASE

Breathing might seem like a simple task, but most people don't know how to breathe to help relieve stress. The first step is to be aware of your breathing. You can follow this simple breath work practice anytime and anywhere.

▸ Sit in a relaxing position with your eyes closed.

▸ Place one hand on your chest and the other on your lower abdomen.

▸ For five to ten minutes, just focus on your breath, noticing your inhalation and your exhalation. As you inhale, allow your lower abdomen to swell like a balloon.

▸ With each breath out, practice relaxing your jaw and shoulders. If your mind wanders, bring your focus back to your breath.

FORGIVENESS WRITING EXERCISE

It's human nature to judge and be judged, develop resentments, and project our issues onto others. These thoughts do not serve us well, and they hold us back from healing. This exercise can help you release judgments, resentments, and built-up emotions. If something or someone upsets you, remember, there's room for healing and forgiveness.

- On a blank sheet of loose-leaf paper (not in a bound journal), freely write down your negative thoughts, judgments, and feelings. Use as many sheets of paper as you need. Whatever comes up, write it down.

- Do *not* read what you've written.

- When you feel there is nothing left to write, burn or shred the papers and throw them away.

- In your journal, or on a separate piece of paper, write down one or more sentences of forgiveness and gratitude.

TEN-MINUTE MEDITATION

Research suggests that meditation helps lower stress, increases our compassion, improves sleep, boosts mood, decreases inflammation, and even helps lowers yearly medical costs. The goal of meditation is to focus and quiet your mind to achieve greater clarity and inner calm. Try this simple ten-minute meditation.

- Choose a quiet place, and turn off any electronics.

- Sit in a relaxing position (but not one that's *too* comfortable—this is not naptime).

- Focus on a word, such as "peace" or "gratitude"—a mantra of sorts—or music or an object, such as a candle.

- When your mind wanders, gently bring your attention back to your focal point.

- If you have limited time, set an alarm so you don't worry about checking the time.

- Let go of expectations. You may or may not have an epiphany.

RELAXING BEDTIME RITUAL

Sleep is essential to help energize us, manage stress, and keep us focused and positive. Ideally, we all should get about eight hours of uninterrupted sleep each night. Create your own relaxing bedtime ritual with any of the following:

- Listen to soothing music.

- Take a warm Mineral Bath (page 91).

- Do gentle yoga or stretches.

- Perform breathing or other relaxation exercises (see page 94).

GRATITUDE JOURNAL

Gratitude is about appreciating what you have around you. Research shows that gratitude helps us feel happier, deal better with problems that arise, and build solid relationships, as well as improves our health. You can practice gratitude in your mind or say it aloud, such as during a prayer or a blessing. My favorite way to anchor in and reap the rewards of gratitude is to keep a gratitude journal. I write down at least one thing every day that I am grateful for.

NATURE EXCURSION

Step away from your computer, phone, or any energy-zapping scenario, and escape into nature. Even if it's just a quick walk around the block, a few moments in the sun and fresh air can boost your mood and give you a little extra vitamin D to brighten your day. It also involves movement, and studies show that moderate exercise improves our energy, mood, and sleep.

A FINAL NOTE

In addition to these techniques, I encourage you to laugh, love, and breathe well for stress release and a clean mind, which can keep you on track for achieving clean skin. All of these practices help balance our hormones and neurotransmitters, such as cortisol, serotonin, and dopamine; create a sense of calm; and restore our health. Reducing cortisol helps reduce skinflammation; and because our hormones are intricately connected, this effect can help balance other hormones related to healthy, glowing skin. With the boost of dopamine and serotonin, our mood improves, and we're more likely to continue healthy lifestyle practices, follow our goals, and achieve greater confidence.

Now that you know the four parts to this program—clean plate, clean slate, clean body, and clean mind—let's put them all together.

If you haven't already, this is a good time to determine your primary skin type. Go to TheSkinQuiz.com before moving on to the next chapter.

CHAPTER 6

Personalizing Your 2-Week Plan

In the previous chapters, I introduced you to the four aspects of my two-week program. The closer you follow the plan, the greater your potential results for clean skin from within. Many people notice a difference in their skin and overall vitality within just a few days. These changes usually continue to improve over the two-week period. For most, this two-week commitment is sufficient to reset the body and achieve radiant skin.

PREPARING FOR THE 2-WEEK PROGRAM

▸ Write down a plan that includes menus, shopping lists, and meal schedules.

▸ If you are constipated, one of your main paths for eliminating waste and toxins is closed. Get regular—take a vitamin C and magnesium supplement, and consider an herbal tea or laxative to help.

▸ Wean yourself off caffeine and sugar.

▸ Do not overindulge before beginning the program. You won't be eliminating these foods forever—just two weeks.

▸ If you have an eating disorder or emotional issues around eating, discuss this program with your doctor before trying it.

Once you've completed your two weeks, optimize your results with the diet, skin care, and lifestyle tips in chapter 10. To review, here are the aspects of my two-week plan.

CLEAN PLATE

Follow the recommendations in chapter 3 and the recipes in chapters 7 (for drinks) and 8 (for food) for the entire two weeks.

Avoid skinflammation-triggering foods; instead, eat foods rich in:

▸ Antioxidants

▸ Cleansing and anti-inflammatory properties

▸ Collagen-boosting nutrients

▸ Prebiotics and probiotics

▸ Skin-loving fatty acids

Get the appropriate number of recommended servings of each of the following food categories (see page 54 for recommended serving sizes):

FOOD	DAILY SERVINGS
Vegetables	6 or more
Fruit	"Sweet" fruit: 1 to 3 servings, plus ½ to 1 avocado or 3 to 6 olives
Clean animal protein	1 to 3 (vegetarians/vegans = 0)
Nuts and seeds	1 to 2 (vegetarians/vegans = 2)
Legumes (beans and peas)	1 to 3 (vegetarians/vegans = 2 to 3)
Gluten-free grains	0 to 1
Fermented foods	1 to 2
Oils	Varies based on other natural fat you consume; if you eat the recommended amounts of the other foods, consume an extra 4 to 6 servings of oils (vegetarians/vegans = 6).
Herbs and spices	At least 2
Liquids	6 or more

Avoid these foods and drinks—listed in order of importance—as much as possible:

1. Sugar
2. Dairy
3. Gluten-containing grains
4. Alcohol
5. Caffeine
6. Eggs
7. Corn
8. Nightshades
9. Peanuts
10. Soy

CLEAN SLATE

Follow the recommendations in chapter 4 and the recipes for DIY skin care in chapter 9.

Avoid the twenty harmful ingredients discussed on pages 77–79 and instead choose natural skin care alternatives that contain healthier fragrances, natural preservatives, nontoxic oils, and plant-based skin-soothers.

Look for natural skin care products with essential oils, including my favorite six essential oils for skin (see pages 81–82), or incorporate them into your DIY recipes.

You'll also use natural ingredients from your kitchen (see page 172), plant-based skin soothers (see page 173), and natural oils such as avocado, coconut, sunflower seed, sweet almond, and jojoba in your DIY skin care regimen.

CLEAN BODY

Follow the recommendations in chapter 5.

Reduce toxins in your home, water, and food (see pages 87–90), and enhance your body's natural detoxification pathways with the home spa cleansing techniques (see pages 90–93).

AN IMPORTANT NOTE FOR PEOPLE WITH CHRONIC SKIN PROBLEMS

If you have a chronic skin condition, you may need to continue this program for an additional two weeks for best results. It takes about thirty days for skin cells to turn over, and you may need that extra time for your skin to heal and revitalize. If you see some improvement at the end of the two-week program but your skin is not fully clear and glowing, repeat the full program.

CLEAN MIND

Follow the recommendations in chapter 5.

Relieve stress and emotional upset that can contribute to skin and other health issues using the practices on pages 93 to 96. I recommend doing at least one of these practices daily during the two-week program. For even greater stress relief, try each practice at least once during the program to determine which works best for you. Notice what happens to your body, as well as your mind, during each, and continue practicing your favorite(s) accordingly.

PERSONALIZING THE PROGRAM BASED ON YOUR SKIN TYPE

Let's consider the five skin types (Amber, Olivia, Heath, Emmett, Sage) and modifications for each during the two-week program.

AMBER

If you're an Amber-type (pages 23–25), your root causes are oxidative damage and hormonal imbalances. During the program, it's crucial to avoid toxins that can enhance oxidative damage. Instead focus on antioxidant-rich and anti-inflammatory foods—in particular, colorful fruits and vegetables.

HORMONAL ISSUES

To address hormonal imbalances, focus on reducing stress, balancing the cortisol that can trigger inflammation and oxidative damage. You may also want to take an adaptogenic herbal formula, such as one containing any or all of the following: ashwagandha, astragalus, ginseng, and rhodiola. Because B vitamins can help regulate the body's stress response, eat food rich in B vitamins, such as free-range chicken, grass-fed beef, and fish. If you're vegan or need additional support, consider taking a B-complex supplement.

Following the clean slate recommendations (see pages 72–80) will help reduce oxidative damage and the possible hormone-disrupting effects of toxic skin care ingredients. Clean body practices (see pages 87–93) will aid your detoxification pathways to balance hormones and reduce oxidative damage.

Pregnancy alert: If you are pregnant, talk with your doctor before starting any supplements. Pregnancy is not a good time to

AMBER SKIN TYPE

Features of the Amber skin type include any or all of the following:

- Hyperpigmentation (darkening or excess pigmentation in certain skin areas)
- Freckles
- Melasma
- Uneven skin tone

do any kind of liver cleansing because it may affect your developing baby.

MELASMA

If you've been coping with melasma as a result of birth control pills, hormone therapy, or pregnancy, the natural cleansing in this program should help. Because your liver plays a key role in hormone metabolism and balance, consider a liver cleanse supplement, such as one containing milk thistle, amino acids, dandelion, and green tea.

Since hyperpigmentation takes time to fade, you may not see a significant difference in just two weeks; the change may be gradual. However, I have seen patients' skin tone begin to even as quickly as two to four weeks. I suggest you take a "before" picture when you start the program as a reference point.

SUPPLEMENTAL SUPPORT FOR AMBER

While nutritional deficiencies may not be your root cause, micronutrients play a key role in oxidative damage. Consider taking supplements, such as omega-3s, and antioxidant and cleansing support formulas. The following table summarizes some specific recommendations.

VITAMINS AND SUPPLEMENTS	TOPICAL TREATMENTS
Astaxanthin Part of the carotenoid family, this potent antioxidant can protect skin from harmful effects of oxidative damage. Aids in skin moisture levels, smoothness, elasticity, and spots or freckles; penetrates skin cells and reduces UVA damage; found in crabs, crayfish, krill, lobster, salmon, shrimp, and trout.	**Nicotinamide gel** 2% to 5%, alone or in combination with N-acetyl glucosamine, can help reduce hyperpigmentation and melasma. A 2010 study in the *British Journal of Dermatology* found topical 2% N-acetyl glucosamine and 4% nicotinamide gel significantly reduced hyperpigmentation in about 200 patients; also appears to decrease inflammation on skin and improve the skin barrier.
Vitamin C Essential for overall health; enhances collagen production and provides skin-brightening benefits.	**Tea** White, green, black, and chamomile teas have great antioxidant, nourishing, and skin-evening effects. Try the Tea Toner (page 181) to ease hyperpigmented or sun-damaged skin.
Vitamin E Antioxidant with skin-softening benefits. Look for mixed tocopherols/tocotrienols on the label, which is closer to what you find in nature.	**Turmeric** Offers beautiful skin-brightening and antioxidant effects; use it carefully to avoid staining your skin. Try the Turmeric-Chickpea Face Mask (page 186).
Vitamin B$_{12}$ B vitamins are essential for healthy skin; B$_{12}$ may be particularly important for Amber-types, as some clinical cases have linked a deficiency with hyperpigmentation.	**Licorice** A 2000 study in the *International Journal of Dermatology* found the active constituent of licorice, liquiritin, helped lighten study participants' skin when applied twice daily as a cream for four weeks. Licorice extract contains other important active naturals that can help even skin tone, so it's easy to find in skin care products.
Pycnogenol Known for its antioxidant properties and ability to protect against UV radiation damage. A 2002 study in the journal *Phytotherapy Research* studied 30 women with melasma. Each took one 25-mg pycnogenol tablet with meals three times daily. After 30 days, melasma intensity and areas affected significantly decreased.	**Green algae (*Chlorella vulgaris*)** Due to high levels of chlorophyll, it shields the body from UV radiation and may protect against sun-related skin changes.
Vitamin D$_3$ Protects skin against oxidative damage.	**Pomegranate seed oil** Rich in the antioxidants ellagic acid, anthocyanins, and the rare omega-5 essential fatty acid; known to even skin tone and prevent oxidative damage.
Adaptogenic herbs Take any or all of the following to address hormonal imbalances: ashwagandha, astragalus, ginseng, and rhodiola.	

OLIVIA

If you're an Olivia-type, blood sugar issues, hormonal imbalances, microbiome disturbances, and inflammation are your root causes. The two-week program addresses all of these underlying triggers. Olivia-types who struggle with acne are not alone—acne affects more than 40 million people. Although sometimes viewed as a superficial health concern, those of us with acne know it can cause permanent damage—both physical and emotional.

According to conventional dermatology, acne occurs when oil from our pores combines with dead skin and clogs the pores. The oil secretions (sebum) build up beneath a blocked pore, allowing bacteria such as *Propionibacterium acnes* (*P. acnes*) to proliferate, causing a breakout. This may be the physiologic change, but what's *really* causing this? The root causes are what separate the occasional breakout from the recurring acne with which many Olivia-types struggle.

BLOOD SUGAR

As you may recall, elevated blood sugar causes insulin to increase, which triggers sebum production. That process can lead to clogged pores and acne. Part of why that happens has to do with genetics and whether your body helps properly regulate your blood sugar. Olivia-types should pay particular attention to their blood sugar and eat foods that keep blood sugar in check. Eating balanced macronutrient (fat, carbohydrate, and protein) proportions and not skipping meals or overindulging in sweets is key. Refer to chapter 2 for recommendations on blood sugar testing and additional dietary modifications.

HORMONAL IMBALANCE

We know increased insulin triggers androgen activity, which brings me to the next root cause for Olivia-types: hormonal imbalances. Excess androgen or testosterone can trigger acne because it increases sebum production. Although this hormonal factor would seem to play a role only during puberty, acne often occurs in female adults as well. More than four out of five people between the ages of twelve and twenty-four develop acne at least once in their life, but over half of the 40 million people with acne are women older than

OLIVIA SKIN TYPE

Features of the Olivia skin type include any or all of the following:

▸ Acne

▸ Large pores

▸ Blackheads

▸ Whiteheads

▸ Sebaceous hyperplasia

age twenty-five. Hormone balance is a key goal for Olivia-types.

Birth control pills are often prescribed to teens and women with acne because of their androgen-suppressing effects. I don't think this is the best approach. Birth control pills suppress and disrupt our innate hormone production, leading to further imbalances. In addition, long-term use of birth control pills can deplete the body of important nutrients, such as riboflavin, pyridoxine, folate, vitamins B12, C, and E, as well as magnesium, selenium, and zinc.

Spironolactone (and other androgen receptor blockers) is another popular treatment for hormonal acne. Its downside is similar because it suppresses androgens and leads to hormonal imbalances. Some women taking this drug experience irregular menstrual cycles, breast tenderness, fatigue, headaches, and melasma, among other symptoms.

It's important to remember that our hormones work together. Stress hormones, for example, greatly affect androgen activity. Clean mind practices can help reduce stress and balance hormones. Clean plate, clean slate, and clean body practices help too. You'll find recommendations in chapters 3,

4, and 5. The clean plate diet includes high fiber, omega-3s, and cruciferous vegetables to support healthy hormone metabolism and balance.

GUT AND SKIN MICROBIOME

As already noted, acne is linked to bacterial overgrowth on the skin, which brings me to another root cause for Olivia-types: microbiome disturbances. This disruption can occur both internally and externally. In general, fermented foods and other microbiome-enhancing foods can help rebalance your gut and skin from within. Refer to chapter 2 for recommendations concerning their importance in supporting the gut microbiome (which also affects the skin microbiome) and how skin care pH affects the latter.

INFLAMMATION

When we have internal inflammation, it appears on the skin (skinflammation); for Olivia-types, it shows up as acne and sebaceous hyperplasia. Avoiding inflammatory triggers can help you reap the rewards of a clean plate, a clean slate, and a clean body.

SUPPLEMENTAL SUPPORT FOR OLIVIA

In addition to the previous recommendations, my favorite supplements for Olivia-types are summarized in the following table. These additional recommendations are designed to support the program, but are optional.

As with all skin types, it's important to have a regular skin care routine with mildly acidic products to create a healthy skin microbiome. Using this type of product to prevent overgrowth of the wrong bacteria is especially important for Olivia-types.

VITAMINS AND SUPPLEMENTS	TOPICAL TREATMENTS
Gamma-linolenic acid (GLA) Studies suggest that evening primrose, black current, and borage oils, which contain GLA, help keep breakouts at bay. They reduce prostaglandin and leukotriene levels, which decrease inflammation. They also help keep hormones that activate skin's oil production under control.	**Tea tree essential oil** Using certain essential oils, such as tea tree, can help reduce breakouts. Essential oils should be diluted when applied to skin.
Omega-3s These fatty acids, such as those in fish oil supplements, are one of my favorite supplements to help decrease inflammation associated with acne.	**Nicotinamide gel** A 2013 paper published in the *International Journal of Dermatology* suggests that topical 4% nicotinamide gel applied twice daily for two months helped significantly reduce acne; appears to reduce excess sebum, decrease skinflammation, and improve the skin barrier.
Zinc Studies show a distinct correlation between low levels of zinc and acne's severity. Zinc reduces inflammation and calms androgens, the hormones that often trigger acne. Take 30 to 60 mg of an oral zinc supplement daily, with 1 to 2 mg of copper and other minerals for balanced nutrition.	**Licorice extract** Can help reduce breakouts; possesses antimicrobial, anti-inflammatory, antihistamine, and sebum-reducing effects.

(continued)

VITAMINS AND SUPPLEMENTS	TOPICAL TREATMENTS
Probiotics These bacteria help keep our gut healthy—particularly important if you take antibiotics for acne. Research indicates that the gut microbiome—the balance of good bacteria—is important to address acne; probiotics can help restore healthy gut flora.	**Yogurt** Applied topically, yogurt may help rebalance the skin microbiome and ward off acne-triggering bacteria. The lactic acid has a sebum-balancing effect. See chapter 9 for DIY skin care ideas.
Curcumin Research shows curcumin has potent antioxidant and anti-inflammatory effects and can greatly decrease acne-triggering bacteria.	**French green clay or bentonite clay** Contains astringent and drawing properties to extract impurities from skin. Avoid drying. See chapter 9.
Glutathione-promoters The level of the antioxidant glutathione is lower in acne sufferers' skin compared with people who don't have acne. Glutathione has powerful antioxidant and detoxification properties. Certain supplements, such as green tea, N-acetyl cysteine, and vitamin C, can boost glutathione levels.	**Aloe** Its soothing, anti-inflammatory, and healing properties makes aloe an ideal ingredient in skin care for acne-prone Olivia-types.
Vitex (chasteberry) Can be helpful when hormonal imbalance is the underlying trigger for skin problems; its hormonal effects are thought to be similar to progesterone's, and research suggests that vitex can relieve acne symptoms.	**Teas (rooibos, black, green, and white)** Anti-inflammatory, antioxidant-rich, and balancing, these can help soothe and clear skin.
Multivitamins and minerals I recommend a high-quality multivitamin and mineral supplement containing B vitamins (preferably in "methyl" form), selenium, chromium, magnesium, vitamin A (mixed carotenoids and beta-carotene), vitamin E (mixed tocopherols), and vitamin D3.	**Turmeric (*Curcuma longa*)** Helps control microorganism growth on the skin, warding off acne-causing *P. acnes* bacteria. It also balances sebum secretion and cleans out pores.

HEATH

The root causes that trigger Heath-types are inflammation, microbiome disturbance, and hormonal imbalance. Whether you have rosacea, visible blood vessels, redness, or just sensitive skin, the two-week program is designed to address your underlying causes and soothe your skin from within.

INFLAMMATION

One of the biggest skin concerns with this skin type is rosacea, which presents as redness, small visible blood vessels, and eruptions on the nose, cheeks, and forehead. If you have this condition, you're not alone—it's estimated to affect more than 16 million Americans, and most don't even know it. In addition to being a hindrance, if untreated, the problem can get worse, even leading to ocular rosacea with burning, red eyes.

Research suggests a genetic component to rosacea because it tends to run in families, especially those of Celtic and Northern European decent (like me!). The condition can worsen with spicy foods, alcohol, caffeine, excess sun exposure, stress, or exercise.

With Heath-types, avoiding inflammatory triggers and incorporating a clean plate, slate, and body are essential to address the root causes. Because stress and cortisol play a role in inflammation and hormone balance, the clean-mind practices are also important.

GUT AND SKIN MICROBIOMES

While characteristics of Heath-types are not associated with bacterial overgrowth on the skin like acne is, maintaining a healthy skin pH and microbiome is still imperative. Doing so helps reduce inflammation externally. Heath-types have very sensitive skin, so it's essential to follow the clean slate and use the DIY skin care recipes in chapter 9. If you have digestive symptoms, such as gas, bloating, heartburn, constipation, diarrhea, or irregular bowel movements, consider adding a probiotic supplement.

SUPPLEMENTAL SUPPORT FOR HEATH

Some supplements recommended for Olivia-types (see table, pages 103–104) are also helpful for Heath-types. For example, after taking GLAs, black currant oil, and evening primrose oil for two weeks, people with rosacea usually show some improvement, which will continue over the next four weeks.

Interestingly, typical Ayurvedic (a form of holistic healing) spices, such as turmeric

HEATH SKIN TYPE

Features of the Heath skin type include any or all of the following:

▸ Easily flushed skin

▸ Reactions to weather or temperature changes

▸ Redness or inflammation, possibly a bumpy texture

▸ Rosacea: redness on face, cheeks, forehead, or chin; may have acne-like bumps

▸ Sensitive skin that reacts easily to skin care products

▸ Telangiectasia (visible blood vessels)

and ginger, do not aggravate rosacea, while other spices do. In fact, adaptogenic Ayurvedic herbs and dietary choices are particularly helpful for rosacea and other Heath-type characteristics. The following table summarizes additional suggestions.

SOOTHING HERBS FOR CLEAN PLATE MEALS	TOPICAL TREATMENTS
Basil	**Nicotinamide** Research suggests nicotinamide topical gel or cream can promote skin health. For Heath-types, it appears to decrease inflammation and irritation.
Ginger	**Oats** Enjoy these for breakfast AND apply them topically to reduce inflammation and nourish skin. Try the Oat, Green Tea, and Yogurt Face Mask (page 186).

(continued)

SOOTHING HERBS FOR CLEAN PLATE MEALS	TOPICAL TREATMENTS
Oregano	**Aloe vera gel** Known for its ability to soothe sensitive, inflamed skin; avoid buying it commercially because it usually contains preservatives, other gels, and ingredients that may compromise its benefits. Choose a pure source from a local health food store, or make your own.
Rosemary	**Green tea** Rich in antioxidants that can soothe and nourish skin. Brew the tea, cool it, then apply to the skin. See chapter 9 for additional suggestions.
Thyme	**MSM and silymarin** Combination MSM and silymarin can help manage symptoms of rosacea, such as stinging, redness, and bumps, according to a report in the March 2008 *Journal of Cosmetic Dermatology*.
Turmeric	**Feverfew** Known to have anti-inflammatory, anti-irritant, and antioxidant properties. Topical application has been shown to reduce skin redness, according to a report, "Cosmetic Benefits of Natural Ingredients," in the September 2014 issue of *Journal of Drugs in Dermatology*.

EMMETT

The immune system—particularly when it's imbalanced—is the connecting factor with this long list of skin issues. Typically, this imbalance occurs because the immune system is overactive, but it may also be underactive. Why does the immune system not respond properly for Emmett-types? The answer lies in the root causes: inflammation, microbiome disturbance, and hormonal imbalance. When you address these, the immune system can return to normal, even optimal, function. This may take more than two weeks for the full effect, but the two-week program can jump-start the process. For long-term benefits, it is important to address the root causes.

Even if you haven't been diagnosed with eczema or psoriasis, as many Emmett-types have been, you may notice you have lost pigmentation (vitiligo) or your skin is itchy, scaly, or dry. These symptoms can all be traced back to the root causes.

GUT AND SKIN MICROBIOME

When our immune system is debilitated due to genetics, poor diet, or other lifestyle factors, we are more likely to develop imbalances in our gut and skin microbiomes. Keeping the immune and digestive systems in proper order is essential for addressing symptoms of Emmett-types.

Most people see results with a digestive-focused plan—one that specifically helps heal a leaky gut and addresses gut microbiome disturbances. Therefore, the diet recommendations within the two-week program, as well as the ongoing recommendations in chapter 10, are extremely beneficial for

EMMETT SKIN TYPE

Features of the Emmett skin type include any or all of the following:

- Allergic skin reactions, such as hives or contact dermatitis

- Atopic dermatitis (often called eczema, which appears as dry, scaly, and, often, itchy, red skin)

- Chronic itching

- Dry, scaly skin

- Keloids (a raised scar that often appears smooth, pink, or purple that can extend beyond the wound site and doesn't improve over time)

- Psoriasis (raised reddish or silver-white scaly patches)

- Recurring acute skin issues and infections, such as impetigo, ringworm, and cold sores

- Seborrheic dermatitis (redness or swelling with white or yellowish scaling of skin, usually in the center of the face, eyebrows, scalp, and ears)

- Vitiligo (patches of lighter skin, or depigmentation)

Emmett-types. To help repair the gut, I suggest consuming collagen-rich foods, such as bone broth, and fermented foods, including dairy-free yogurts, drinks, and kimchi.

INFLAMMATION

When our immune system is overactive, we are more likely to develop allergies and autoimmune diseases that can affect the skin. Stress and irritants, such as soaps, allergens, and climate, often trigger Emmett-types' symptoms too.

A June 2007 study published in *Dermatitis* suggested that nearly 32 million people in the United States have the most common skin problem for this type: eczema. Psoriasis is another common skin condition among Emmett-types. About 7.4 million American adults were affected by psoriasis in 2013, according to a March 2014 study published in the *Journal of the American Academy of Dermatology.*

The two-week plan will help eczema sufferers because it addresses inflammation, heals the gut, and offers the immune system a break. For Emmett-types, one of the most valuable takeaways from completing the two-week program will reveal itself after the program ends. In chapter 10 you will learn how to reintroduce eliminated foods to your diet and learn which may trigger your symptoms. Avoiding your triggers long term gives your digestive tract a chance to heal.

SUPPLEMENTAL SUPPORT FOR EMMETT

If you're like Emmett, you may need supplements to further address the underlying causes. The following table summarizes additional suggestions for Emmett-types that I have found support the immune system and GI tract while helping decrease inflammation.

VITAMINS AND SUPPLEMENTS	TOPICAL TREATMENTS
Probiotics Research suggests that probiotics help the immune response, enhance the gut microbiome, and help reduce eczema.	**Nicotinamide gel** This treatment, in gel or cream form, has anti-inflammatory properties that appear to help relieve atopic dermatitis.
Essential fatty acids (EFAs) Omega-3s and evening primrose oil are excellent choices for their anti-inflammatory properties.	**Green tea** Antioxidant and anti-inflammatory properties make green tea, as well as white tea, another top pick for Emmett-types.
Vitamin D3 Its immune-modulating effects make it a great option. Have your blood levels tested to determine how much your body needs.	**Vitamin B12** Topically applied, it appears to decrease inflammation for some.
Zinc Research suggests individuals with low zinc levels can find relief from skinflammation and itching by taking this supplement.	**Coconut oil** Extremely hydrating and appears to control common bacteria on the skin, such as staph.
Multivitamin and mineral supplement I recommend a high-quality multivitamin and mineral supplement to help support skin repair and decrease inflammation.	**Licorice gel** *Glycyrrhiza glabra* standardized extract is known for its anti-inflammatory effects. In one study, 2% licorice topical gel helped reduce redness, swelling, and itching over two weeks in eczema patients.
Homeopathic remedies A few top choices are sulfur, graphites, rhus tox, and arsenicum. Choose a 12C, 30C, or X potency; opt for the one best suited for your skin condition, or work with a homeopathic practitioner.	**Diluted apple cider vinegar soaks** Known for its pH-balancing effects; diluted apple cider vinegar can soothe irritated skin and help restore balance to help it heal.
Chinese medicine Chinese herbs and acupuncture have been known to help decrease irritation, inflammation, and itchy skin. See a licensed acupuncturist or Chinese medicine practitioner for support.	**Oatmeal bath** Colloidal oatmeal in skin care products soothes and moisturizes itchy, inflamed skin. See preparation instructions on page 192 for full-body relief.
	Aloe vera Its soothing, healing properties can help repair inflamed skin.
	Calendula High levels of flavonoids, triterpene saponins, and carotenoids provide anti-inflammatory and antimicrobial effects to help skin heal.
	St. John's wort Topical creams with this anti-inflammatory, antibacterial ingredient can improve skin.
	Chamomile One trial reported in *Methods and Findings in Experimental and Clinical Pharmacology* found chamomile to be about 60% as effective as 0.25% hydrocortisone cream in treating eczema. Because it is part of the ragweed family, anyone with a ragweed allergy should do a patch test first.

SAGE

As we age, our skin changes, so its appearance evolves as well. Our skin becomes thinner and more fragile. This process is natural, and there's nothing wrong with aging. But we can take certain steps to help protect, enhance, and nourish skin as it grows older with our bodies. Sage-types' root causes are oxidative damage, blood sugar issues, hormonal imbalances, and nutritional deficiencies. The two-week program will address all of these so you can age gracefully.

With Sage-types, it's important to reduce triggers for oxidative damage and repair the body with antioxidant-rich foods and skin care. Antioxidant supplements can also help. Blood sugar imbalances trigger oxidative damage—another reason to eliminate sugar and eat balanced meals.

It's also a good idea to have your fasting blood sugar and HbA1C levels tested to see if blood sugar imbalance is a particular issue for you. When you have that blood work done, have your doctor check your vitamin D and hormone levels too. They can play a huge role in skin changes for Sage-types. Knowing your unique issues can really help customize your two-week program and ongoing approach to skin care.

Nutritional deficiencies are common as time passes. Sage-types need to be partic-

ularly attentive to their diet. Eat nutrient-dense foods and consider supplements to support overall health and glowing skin.

SUPPLEMENTAL SUPPORT FOR SAGE

Sage-types can slow signs of aging by following these recommendations. I encourage you to take a picture before the two-week program. Fine lines appear or disappear often without us knowing, and it's often hard to monitor these changes without a picture to compare. Most Sage-types will need at least four weeks before seeing significant changes, but you might notice changes as early as the end of the two-week program. The following tables summarize key supplements for Sage-types:

VITAMINS AND SUPPLEMENTS	TOPICAL TREATMENTS
Collagen Production naturally depletes as we age, especially after age 40. Consider taking a high-quality collagen supplement from a clean source.	**Nicotinamide** Increases collagen synthesis and that of other proteins to help moisturize skin and keep it elastic. A 2005 study published in the journal *Dermatologic Surgery* showed 5% nicotinamide cream applied to the face for 12 weeks led to a significant reduction in fine lines, wrinkles, age spots, and sallow skin. A 2008 study in the *Journal of Dermatology* suggested 4% nicotinamide cream decreased wrinkles over eight weeks.

(continued)

VITAMINS AND SUPPLEMENTS	TOPICAL TREATMENTS
Astaxanthin A number of studies show how astaxanthin aids in skin moisture levels, smoothness, and elasticity, which can reduce unwanted fine lines and wrinkles, as well as age spots.	**Vitamin C** Many skin care companies sell vitamin C serums for mature skin; I prefer skin care with naturally occurring vitamin C. Look for ingredients found in nature, such as strawberries and sea buckthorn fruit oil, naturally high in vitamin C. Be careful with citrus-containing ingredients because of their sun-sensitizing effects.
Glutathione enhancers If you have a history of excessive toxin exposure or need a boost with hormone metabolism, consider support to increase glutathione, such as NAC and vitamin C.	**Green tea** Its antioxidant (polyphenols) and nourishing benefits make green tea, as well as white and red teas, a top choice for mature skin.
DIM or Idole-3-Carbinol If you have signs of hormonal imbalance, such as irregular cycles, hormonal acne, or breast tenderness, consider additional hormone metabolism support with DIM or I-3-C.	**Vitamin E** This ingredient is ideal for aging skin because it helps block the lipid peroxidation responsible for cell membrane damage and is a potent free radical scavenger. Use a mixed blend of tocopherols, such as sunflower oil from non-GMO sources, similar to what you find in nature.
Multivitamin or mineral supplement Because of Sage's tendency to have nutritional deficiencies and the fact so many micronutrients (especially antioxidants) are essential for skin, taking a multivitamin and mineral supplement is key. **Probiotics** Shown to reduce water loss and wrinkle depth and improve skin elasticity after taking for 12 weeks.	**Coenzyme Q10** Topical application with CoQ10 improves skin's levels, providing protective antioxidant effects; it may help reduce fine wrinkles around the eyes.
EFAs Both omega-3s and GLAs are important for skin hydration and decrease inflammation from within. A high-quality supplement could include evening primrose oil, krill oil, and omega-3 from fish.	**Resveratrol** Applied to the skin, this antioxidant is linked to antiaging and anti-inflammatory effects. A special resveratrol fermented by *Pichia pastoris* yeast, it has been shown to have a greater degree of hydration and wrinkle-smoothing effects compared to controls.
Vitamin C Because of its role in collagen production, wound repair, and ability to help reverse UV skin damage, this is an essential nutrient for aging skin.	**Sodium hyaluronate** Hyaluronic acid has a high water-binding capacity, so it acts as a hydrating agent and space filler. It also supports collagen and elastin by keeping them nourished and moist and reduces the appearance of wrinkles while keeping skin soft, smooth, and supple.

CHAPTER 7

Skin-Perfecting Smoothies, Juices, and Drinks

Get ready to dive into delicious, easy-to-prepare smoothie and drink recipes that also offer huge benefits for the skin—some even double as beauty treatments! Some recipes feature the absolute top foods for clear skin, such as avocados and coconut, and contain key ingredients that can help fight inflammation and cleanse skin from within.

Making smoothies, as opposed to juicing with raw vegetables, retains all the fiber, as well as other nutrients—two of the main perks of consuming fruits and veggies in the first place. Not only does fiber help us feel full, but it also promotes skin health because it keeps the digestive system in check.

One caveat: *Don't overdo the fruit.* I know fruit is sweet and delicious, and in small quantities it is great for you. But also include nutrient-rich green leafy veggies, such as spinach, kale, or lettuce, in your smoothie when you can.

Choose organic produce as much as possible to avoid pesticide exposure, which can compromise skin health. For a list of the top most-contaminated and least-contaminated fruits and veggies, visit the Environmental Working Group's website: ewg.org.

Starting your morning with a healthy smoothie can set the right tone to make healthy choices throughout the day. By sipping one, you will feel more balanced and energetic, and less likely to fall prey to skin-sabotaging foods that may come your way.

These ingredients may spark ideas for your own smoothie recipes, and you should feel free to make any adjustments to fit your needs and preferences. I've carefully designed the recipes in this chapter, but I know taste preferences vary—and enjoying what you eat is crucial for forming good habits, as well as for your happiness. Regardless of how you approach these recipes, use the best ingredients possible. You will find most (but not all) of these ingredients in the following recipes.

1. Fresh or frozen fruit: apple, avocado (fresh not frozen), berries, cherries, figs (fresh), guava, kiwi, mango, papaya, passion fruit, peaches, pear, watermelon

2. Greens and other veggies: beets, carrots, celery, chard, collard greens, cucumber, kale, lettuce, spinach

3. Liquids: almond milk and coconut milk (unsweetened), hemp milk, fermented coconut water, filtered water, freshly squeezed or pressed juice, herbal teas

4. Lemon juice or lime juice (fresh): include some rind for extra zing

5. Fresh herbs and spices: basil, cilantro, cinnamon, cloves, ginger, mint, nutmeg, parsley, turmeric

6. Protein powder: hemp or pea

7. Seeds, nuts, and nut butters (always use raw, not roasted): chia seeds, coconut, flaxseed, pumpkin seeds, soaked almonds, walnuts or cashews, sunflower seeds

8. Sweeteners and flavor enhancers:

▸ Dates, large, pitted (2 to 4 is enough to sweeten most smoothies): Even though dates contain high amounts of natural sugars, they are actually a low glycemic index food. According to a study in the 2011 issue of *Nutrition Journal*, they did not significantly raise blood sugar levels after being eaten. According to the USDA's National Nutrient Database, one pitted date contains 1.6 g of fiber.

▸ Extracts: Vanilla, peppermint, and others; make sure they're organic and contain no hidden ingredients.

▸ Fruit: Bananas, dates, grapes, and pineapple are the sweetest.

▸ Stevia: Use drops, plant leaf, or powder.

▸ Nutrient boosters: collagen, coconut oil, maca, probiotics, spirulina/chlorella (algae), vitamin C

To thicken: Add 1 tablespoon (11 g) chia seeds and let soak in liquid for a few minutes to expand.

To make smoother: Add one-fourth of an avocado, ¼ cup (35 g) of cashews, or ¼ cup (20 g) of coconut flesh.

To cool the temperature: Add ¼ cup (1 g) of ice made from filtered water or ¼ cup (about 60 g) of frozen fruit.

To sweeten: Add 1 to 2 pitted dates, a dash of stevia, ¼ teaspoon cinnamon, or ¼ cup (about 40 g) of pineapple or grapes or one-fourth of a banana.

SMOOTHIE TIPS

▸ Use a high-speed blender, such as a Vitamix or BlendTec (or use a food processor for more fibrous veggies, nuts, seeds, and other items, and then add them to a regular blender).

▸ Prep ahead by soaking nuts in filtered water overnight in your fridge and putting kefir grains in your coconut water on the counter overnight.

▸ Looking for a dessert? Make any smoothie recipe and pour it into a popsicle mold. Freeze overnight for a delicious dessert you can enjoy any time of day.

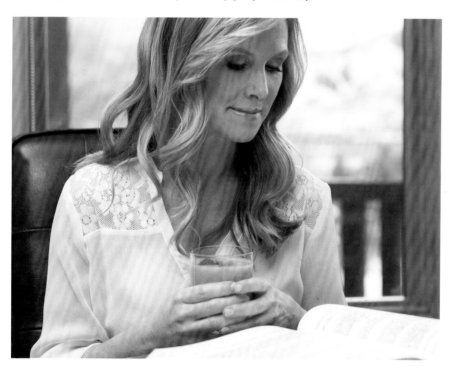

IT'S EASY BEING GREEN >

You may be wary of green-colored drinks, but believe me when I say this refreshing smoothie will go down easy. Pineapple and grapes add just the right amount of sweetness to mask the bitter, nutrient-dense greens, and cilantro and lime add a touch of fresh, clean flavor to this classic.

YIELD: 1 smoothie

1 cup (235 ml) brewed chamomile tea
1 cup (30 g) fresh organic spinach
½ cup (75 g) seedless green grapes
½ cup (42.5 g) pineapple, frozen
¼ medium organic green apple

2 tablespoons (30 g) hemp protein powder
1 teaspoon ground chia seeds
1 teaspoon chopped fresh cilantro
Fresh lime juice, to taste

In a blender, combine all the ingredients and blend until smooth. Pour into a tall glass and enjoy cold.

CREAMY PAPAYA SMOOTHIE

Papaya is a powerful healthy-skin-from-within food, and this creamy, dreamy recipe is just one way to reap its benefits. Cashews give this formula its thick texture, while ginger offers an extra kick—plus antioxidants and digestion-aiding perks.

YIELD: 1 smoothie

1¼ cups (295 ml) chilled organic
    unsweetened coconut milk
1 cup (55 g) organic lettuce
    (anything except iceberg)
½ cup (70 g) chopped papaya

¼ cup (35 g) raw cashews
¼ cup (1 g) ice made from filtered water
2 pitted dates
1 tablespoon (15 ml) fresh lime juice
¼ teaspoon grated fresh ginger

In a blender, combine all the ingredients and blend until smooth. Pour into a tall glass and enjoy cold.

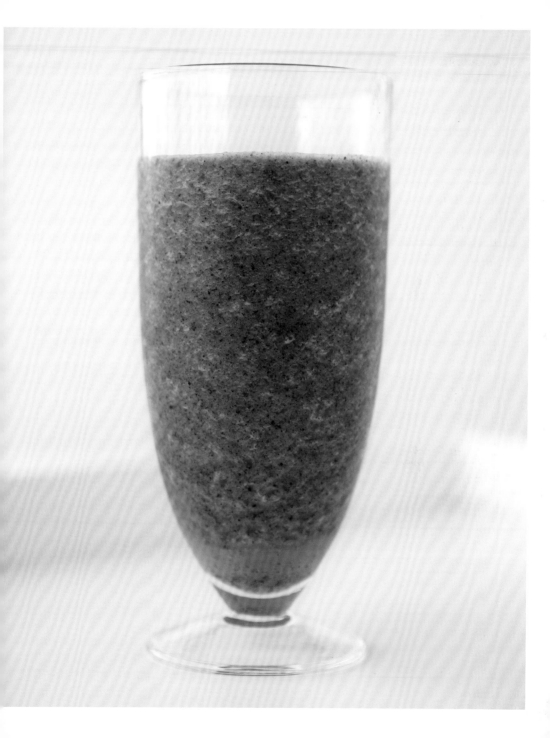

RED VELVET SMOOTHIE

Smooth and luxurious, this red-hued smoothie is not only eye-catching but also tasty. Prepared correctly, avocado adds a creamy texture. (Just don't blend for too long, or its consistency will thicken, resembling mousse.) Beets are rich in vitamin C and fiber and contain betaine, which helps decrease inflammation and supports detoxification.

YIELD: 1 smoothie

1 cup (235 ml) organic unsweetened almond milk
½ cup (112.5 g) peeled, sliced raw beet
½ cup (77.5 g) frozen cherries
¼ avocado

1 tablespoon (12 g) flaxseed
1 teaspoon fresh lime juice
¼ teaspoon pure vanilla extract

In a blender, combine all the ingredients and blend until smooth. Pour into a tall glass and enjoy cold.

BACK TO YOUR ROOTS SMOOTHIE

Cooler fall and winter weather makes the perfect time to enjoy this comforting smoothie. Seasonally fresh root vegetables, full of antioxidants, and ginger help warm the body despite the beverage's cool temperature. If you're not a fan of ginger, try to acquire a taste for it. This powerhouse ingredient contains anti-inflammatory properties and aids digestion.

YIELD: 1 smoothie

1 cup (235 ml) organic unsweetened coconut milk, or unsweetened almond milk
½ cup (112.5 g) peeled, sliced raw beet
½ cup (65 g) chopped carrots
½ cup (50 g) chopped celery

½ cup (85 g) chopped pear
½ cup (75 g) frozen blueberries
¼ cup (36 g) raw almonds soaked in filtered water overnight, drained
¼ teaspoon grated fresh ginger

In a blender, combine all the ingredients and blend until smooth. Pour into a tall glass and enjoy cold.

VERY VEGGIE SMOOTHIE

What better way to start your day than by helping meet your daily vegetable quota with three fresh servings? Apple, fresh herbs, lime juice, and ginger infuse this nutritious formula with a blast of flavor—so much so you won't feel as though you're slurping down a liquid salad. Add extra nourishment with spirulina or chlorella super-greens.

YIELD: 1 smoothie

1 cup (235 ml) organic unsweetened coconut milk
1 cup (71 g) organic mixed greens
½ cup (70 g) chopped cucumber
½ cup (65 g) chopped carrot
½ cup (62.5 g) chopped organic apple
1 tablespoon (6 g) fresh herbs of choice,
    such as mint, cilantro, or parsley

1 tablespoon (11 g) chia seeds
1 tablespoon (7 g) spirulina, or chlorella
    (optional; for extra "green")
1 teaspoon fresh lemon juice, or lime juice
½ teaspoon grated fresh ginger

In a blender, combine all the ingredients, including the spirulina (if using), and blend until smooth. Pour into a tall glass and enjoy cold.

TROPICAL SMOOTHIE

If you're in need a tropical escape, sipping this light, refreshing drink is certain to make you think you've been whisked away to a sunny island. The enzymes in papaya and pineapple aid digestion and help decrease inflammation. Chia seeds help thicken the mixture, and dates and a dash of stevia add a tinge of sweetness. If your papaya and pineapple are super-ripe, skip the dates and stevia.

YIELD: 1 smoothie

1 cup (235 ml) organic unsweetened coconut milk
½ cup (70 g) chopped papaya
¼ avocado
¼ cup (42.5 g) chopped pineapple
¼ cup (21 g) unsweetened organic coconut flakes

2 pitted dates
1 tablespoon (11 g) chia seeds
1 tablespoon (15 ml) fresh lime juice
Handful of ice made from filtered water
Dash of stevia powder

In a blender, combine all the ingredients and blend until smooth. Pour into a tall glass and enjoy cold.

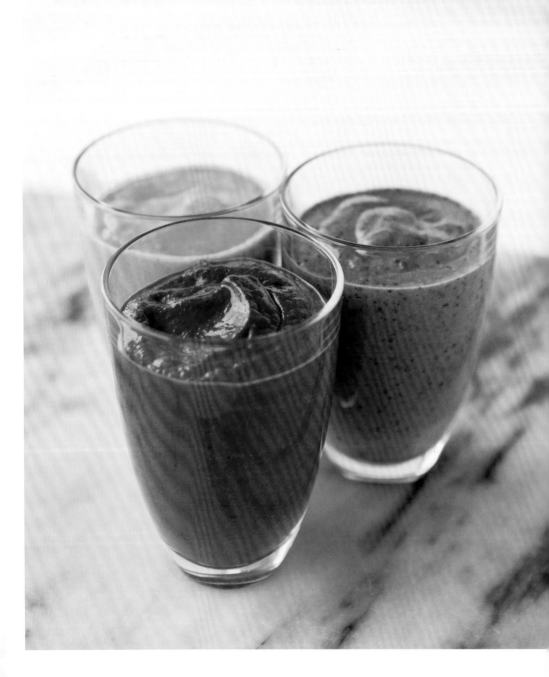

PURPLE PASSION

Simple but bursting with wholesome flavor, this smoothie is packed with antioxidants. Enjoy this beverage any time of year because berries are always available in the freezer section of your grocery store. If you can't find seedless grapes, skip them, but keep in mind the drink won't taste as sweet as the formula listed below.

YIELD: 1 smoothie

1 cup (235 ml) unsweetened rice milk
½ cup (75 g) frozen strawberries
½ cup (77.5 g) frozen blueberries
½ cup (15 g) fresh organic spinach

¼ cup (37.5 g) seedless red grapes
    or purple grapes
1 tablespoon (15 g) unsweetened protein powder

In a blender, combine all the ingredients and blend until smooth. Pour into a tall glass and enjoy cold.

PUMPKIN SMOOTHIE

Pumpkins aren't only a fall decoration—they're a terrific source of beta-carotene, a potent antioxidant that helps protect skin from within. Cinnamon, nutmeg, and ginger make this recipe another festive option for fall or winter.

YIELD: 1 smoothie

1 cup (235 ml) organic unsweetened almond milk
½ cup (122.5 g) canned pure pumpkin,
    or cooked and puréed
½ cup (62.5 g) chopped organic apple
2 pitted dates

1 tablespoon (11 g) chia seeds
1 tablespoon (9 g) raw organic pumpkin seeds
¼ teaspoon ground cinnamon
⅛ teaspoon ground nutmeg
⅛ teaspoon ground ginger, or freshly grated

In a blender, combine all the ingredients and blend until smooth. Pour into a tall glass and enjoy cold.

GOLDEN SMOOTHIE >

Turmeric gives a golden appearance and an anti-inflammatory perk to this deliciously tropical recipe. Maca is an adaptogenic plant belonging to the brassica family; adding it to this smoothie provides extra nourishment and hormone-balancing support.

YIELD: 1 smoothie

1 cup (235 ml) organic unsweetened coconut milk
⅓ cup (28 g) unsweetened organic coconut flakes
⅓ cup (58 g) fresh mango, or frozen
2 pitted dates
1 tablespoon (11 g) chia seeds

1 teaspoon organic virgin coconut oil
½ teaspoon turmeric
½ teaspoon dried maca (optional)
¼ cup (1 g) ice cubes made from filtered water
(omit if using frozen mango)

In a blender, combine all the ingredients, including the maca (if using), and blend until smooth. Pour into a tall glass and enjoy cold.

PEAR GREEN SMOOTHIE

Fresh and yummy, this smoothie is ultra-nourishing, with vitamin C and fiber-rich pears. Be sure to resist peeling the organic apples and pears—the peels are packed with skin- and body-nourishing properties. Soaked overnight, almonds are easier to blend and taste smoother in your smoothies.

YIELD: 1 smoothie

1 cup (30 g) fresh organic spinach
¾ cup (175 ml) organic unsweetened almond milk
½ cup (115 g) chopped pear
½ cup (62.5 g) chopped organic apple
¼ avocado

¼ cup (36 g) raw almonds soaked in filtered
water overnight, drained
1 teaspoon fresh lemon juice
7 mint leaves
¼ to ½ cup (1 to 2 g) ice made from filtered water

In a blender, combine all the ingredients and blend until smooth. Pour into a tall glass and enjoy cold.

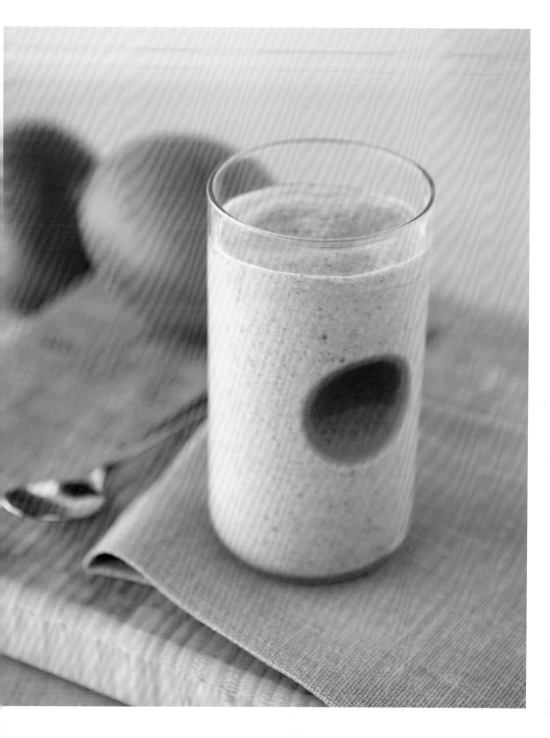

Fresh juices are packed with nutrients—but without the filling fiber—and provide a refreshing option to enjoy throughout the day. There is a huge range of juicers—both in price and type. Choose one that fits your budget.

Avoid juices that have been sitting on a shelf or in a refrigerator for more than two days, because they lose their nutritional value and what mostly remains is the naturally occurring sugar. Choose organic and local ingredients when possible.

Experiment with the following combinations to find your favorite blend, or create one of your own. Note that yields will depend on your juicer. For all of these, process all ingredients through your juicer and serve.

WARMING CARROT

Ideal for fall and winter, when carrots and apples are seasonally available. The ginger helps warm you during cooler weather, and you can add organic greens for extra nourishment.

YIELD: about 1½ cups (355 ml)

5 carrots
1 organic red apple
2 tablespoons (12 g) chopped fresh ginger

GREEN JUICE

This green juice is my favorite because its simple formula perfectly balances nutrient-rich veggies and delicious sweetness from green apple.

YIELD: about 2 cups (473 ml)

4 romaine lettuce leaves, or kale leaves
2 organic green apples
2 ribs celery
½ cucumber

LETTUCE REFRESHER

These veggies contain skin-nourishing nutrients you're sure to feel on the first sip. The carrot and beet add sweetness, and the cucumber adds liquid for a refreshing drink that will help cool you.

YIELD: about 1¾ cups (414 ml)

5 carrots
4 romaine lettuce leaves, or kale leaves
1 beet
½ cucumber

WATERMELON COOLER

This combination makes a refreshing beverage for warm spring and summer days. For added nutrition, add some organic lettuce greens. You can also add 12 mint leaves and the juice of half a lime for a flavor twist. Serve cold, garnished with the mint.

YIELD: about 3 cups (710 ml)

4 cups watermelon flesh
1 large cucumber
1 sprig fresh mint

Save money while nourishing your body by making your own delicious nut milks, mock-tails, and warm beverages. It's easier than you might think! The best part is they're fresh, meaning their nutritional value is higher, and you don't have to worry about hidden sugar and other additives.

ALMOND MILK

Here's another tasty homemade surprise! Fresh almond milk is creamier and tastier than purchased varieties. Make extra, because you may end up drinking it all before you have a chance to add it to your smoothie. For a flavorful horchata-style version, add cinnamon.

YIELD: about 3 cups (710 ml)

1 cup (95 g) raw almonds

3 cups (705 ml) filtered water, plus more for soaking the nuts

½ teaspoon pure vanilla extract (optional)

¼ to ½ teaspoon ground cinnamon, nutmeg, or cloves (optional)

Dash of stevia powder (optional)

Soak the almonds for at least 6 hours, or overnight, in enough water to cover. Drain the water from the almonds and discard it.

In a food processor or high-speed blender, blend the 3 cups (705 ml) of water and the drained almonds until smooth. Strain the blended almonds through a cheesecloth, squeezing out as much liquid as possible. Add the vanilla (if using), spices to taste (if using), and a dash of stevia powder, if desired.

Keeps well in the refrigerator for 3 or 4 days. Enjoy by itself or include it in smoothies.

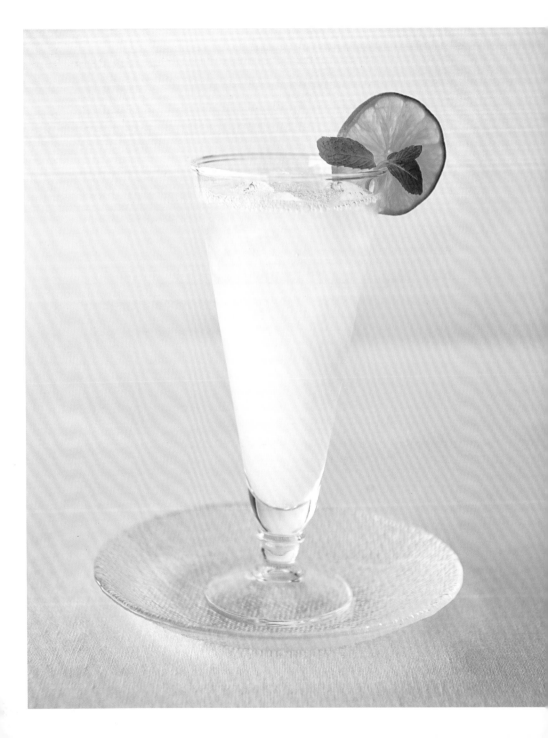

COCO MOCKTAIL FIZZ

Missing those cocktails but want to stay on track? Here's a light, yummy alternative you can enjoy mojito-style with mint. You can even add fresh berries or lime slices for a festive look. Don't be afraid to take this to parties, but bring extra because your friends will want some too!

YIELD: 1 quart (1 L)

4 cups (1 L) unpasteurized coconut water (boxed or fresh from a green coconut)
1 packet (5 g) kefir starter, or 1 teaspoon probiotic powder

1 tablespoon (15 ml) fresh lime juice
Liquid stevia, or coconut palm sugar
1 lime slice
2 sprigs fresh mint, or fresh basil

In a saucepan over medium heat, warm the coconut water to between 92°F and 100°F (33°C and 38°C). Pour it into to a clean 1-liter jar with a swing-top lid. Add the kefir starter. Close the lid and shake well. Place the jar in a dry cooler and let ferment at room temperature for 24 to 36 hours. You will know it's ready when the coconut water starts to bubble and turn cloudy.

Once fermented, add the lime juice and a few drops of liquid stevia, to taste. Pour into a cocktail glass, and garnish with the lime. For a mojito-style drink, macerate the mint in the glass first and then fill with the coconut water. Enjoy cold.

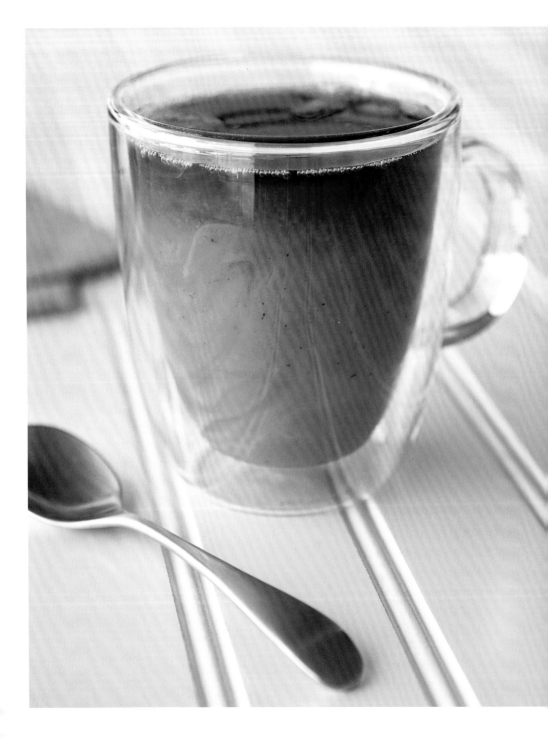

SKIN-NOURISHING COFFEE SUBSTITUTE

Miss your morning cup of coffee? No need to feel deprived with this nourishing, warm drink, but without the overstimulating, dehydrating effects of traditional caffeinated coffee. I use dandelion root with added natural vanilla, but you can add natural vanilla yourself if you like.

YIELD: 6 8-ounce (235 ml) servings

6 cups (1.4 L) filtered water
1 tablespoon (14 g) granulated, roasted dandelion root

1 tablespoon (14 g) granulated, roasted chicory root
1 tablespoon (2 g) rooibos tea
Unsweetened coconut milk (optional)

In a saucepan, boil the water. Place the herbs in a tea ball, or loose in the water, and steep for 5 to 7 minutes. Strain and serve plain or with coconut milk (if using).

RECIPE NOTE   For a richer option, add ½ teaspoon organic virgin coconut oil per cup, or 1 tablespoon (14 g) per pot. For a creamier latte style, combine the tea with ½ teaspoon organic virgin coconut oil per cup and coconut milk, to taste, in a blender. Blend for 5 to 10 seconds. For sweetness, add a dash of stevia powder or ground cinnamon. Serve warm.

COCONUT MILK

Creamy and smooth, you won't be believe how tasty coconut milk can be when made fresh. While I often buy unsweetened coconut milk, I really prefer it homemade. Try it yourself and see!

YIELD: about 2 cups (475 ml)

1 fresh green coconut (available at Asian markets and some health food stores)

1½ cups (355 ml) filtered water

With a machete or end of large kitchen knife (closest to handle), carefully chop a circle around the top of the coconut and peel off the top. This is the hardest part, but with some practice you'll become a pro. Pour the coconut water into a blender; then scoop out the coconut flesh and add it to blender. Add the water and blend until smooth.

Alternatively, if fresh coconut is not available, combine 2 cups of warm filtered water plus 1 cup dry unsweetened shredded coconut in a blender; process until smooth.

Strain the mixture through cheesecloth, squeezing out as much liquid as possible. Repeat straining through cheesecloth to remove extra pulp.

This keeps well in the refrigerator for 3 or 4 days. Enjoy by itself or include it in smoothies.

RECIPE NOTE For additional flavor, add ¼ to ½ teaspoon pure vanilla extract or ground cinnamon, nutmeg, or cloves. For a sweeter taste, add a few drops of liquid stevia or a dash of stevia powder, to taste.

TURMERIC-GINGER COCONUT MILK

This warm, anti-inflammatory beverage is great for a cold day or anytime you want a delicious, comforting treat.

YIELD: 2 8-ounce (235 ml) servings

2 cups (475 ml) organic unsweetened coconut milk

1 teaspoon turmeric

1 teaspoon ground ginger, or freshly grated

Dash pepper

1 teaspoon organic raw honey

1 teaspoon coconut oil

In a saucepan over medium heat, warm the coconut milk. Stir in the turmeric, ginger, and pepper. Simmer, but do not boil, for about 5 minutes. Stir in the honey and coconut oil. Serve warm.

CHAPTER 8

Superfood Recipes for Clean, Glowing Skin

I'm excited to share with you my favorite skin-nourishing and cleansing recipes. Some of the same foods I recommend applying topically to skin are found here. My use of these common ingredients is intentional so that you can recycle unused materials to create DIY face masks after you've whipped up the recipes.

One of my biggest hopes for you is that by following the recipes in this book you'll feel empowered to use whole foods in your diet. Most consumers are so accustomed to packaged convenience foods and fast-food restaurants that we lose sight of the amazing upside home-cooked meals made with fresh, whole ingredients offer—and it does not have to be expensive or time-consuming. In fact, you'll likely save money by switching from processed foods to whole foods you prepare at home.

COOKING WITH CHILDREN

Preparing food at home can instill healthy habits and teach children that fast food isn't the norm. You may discover spending time in the kitchen with your kids, and around the dinner table, offers opportunities to bond over a healthy meal (or even discuss what healthy habits mean to you!). It's important to make the experience around healthful food fun, not restrictive.

If you are visibly following new dietary and lifestyle recommendations, resist the urge to complain in front of your kids. Children pick up on negative comments, and vocalizing your sentiments can profoundly affect their associations with what's on their plate. Instead, if you have negative opinions about food or your body, use the forgiveness writing exercise and journaling (see page 95).

Soups are an easy way to obtain plentiful nutrients all in one bowl as the liquid absorbs the nutrients from the soup ingredients. Enjoy any of these soups or stews alone or with one of the sides or salads. You can also top these soups with fresh herbs or dulse and other seaweed vegetable sprinkles. If you're vegetarian, double the amount of beans to replace the meat in any of these recipes.

THE SPA DR.'S BONE BROTH

Enjoy this bone broth—alone as a snack or drink, or incorporated into other recipes—not only for its taste but also for its skin-enhancing benefits, starting with collagen, crucial for reducing fine lines and wrinkles.

YIELD: about 4 quarts (3.8 L)

2 pounds (905 g) grass-fed beef marrow bones
5 quarts (4.7 L) filtered water
6 carrots, cut into large chunks
5 ribs celery, cut into large chunks
1 medium yellow onion, quartered
1 cup (35 g) shiitake mushrooms
2 tablespoons (30 ml) apple cider vinegar

1-inch (2.5 cm) piece fresh ginger, skin on, halved
1 teaspoon Himalayan salt or Celtic sea salt (or more to taste)
½ bunch fresh Italian parsley, chopped
7 sprigs fresh thyme
6 sprigs fresh rosemary
5 cloves garlic, peeled and crushed or diced

Preheat the oven to 350°F (180°C, or gas mark 4). In a large roasting pan, roast the bones for 30 minutes. (You can skip this step, but it adds nice flavor to the broth.) Transfer to a large (6-quart/5.7 L) soup pot or slow cooker.

Add the water, carrots, celery, onion, mushrooms, cider vinegar, ginger, and salt. Bring to boil; reduce the heat to a very low simmer and cover. Cook for 24 to 48 hours. Skim off any foam that forms on top during the first hour of cooking. The longer you simmer the broth, the more bone marrow nutrients will seep into it.

During the last hour of cooking, stir in the parsley, thyme, rosemary, and garlic. Strain, and enjoy warm, or add to one of the recipes as indicated.

VARIATIONS Instead of beef bones you can use free-range chicken bones (simmer for 12 to 24 hours) or fish bones (simmer for 8 hours). You can use only vegetables if you're vegan or vegetarian; you won't obtain the bone marrow benefits, but you will still obtain nutrients from the vegetables. Skip the bones and add more celery, carrots, broccoli, and other vegetables, such as greens (kale, collard greens, chard), and simmer until the vegetables are tender.

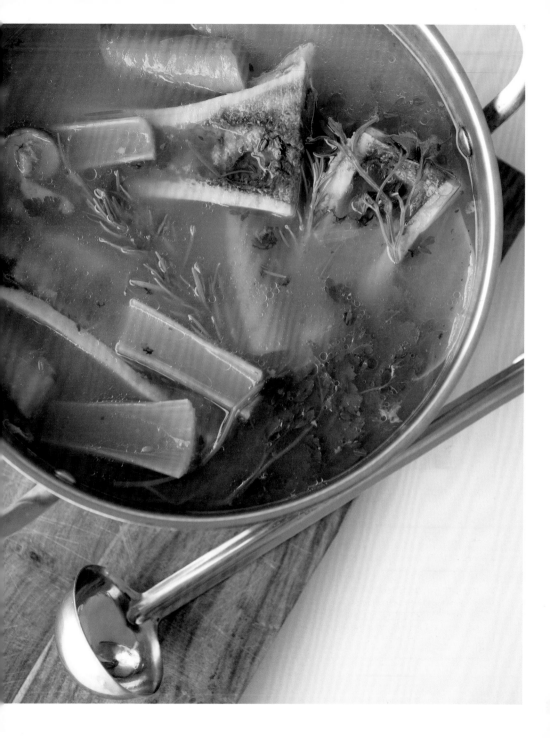

FALL AND WINTER SOUPS AND STEWS

These heartier warm soups are best during the cooler fall and winter months, or when you're feeling chilled and need something to warm you up.

BUTTERNUT SQUASH SOUP

This creamy, savory soup contains butternut squash, rich in fiber and vitamins A and C—let's call it a skin superfood. For a vegan twist on this skin-nourishing recipe, substitute vegetarian broth for the chicken broth.

YIELD: about 6 servings

2 tablespoons (28 g) organic virgin coconut oil

¾ cup (120 g) chopped onion

1 cup (130 g) thinly sliced carrot

½ teaspoon ground cumin

¼ teaspoon ground ginger

¼ teaspoon Himalayan salt or Celtic sea salt (or more to taste)

1 large butternut squash, halved, seeds and pulp removed, peeled, and cut into 1-inch (2.5 cm) pieces

2 cups (475 ml) free-range chicken broth

1 cup (235 ml) organic unsweetened coconut milk

Pepper

Heat the coconut oil in a large soup pot over medium heat. Add the onion and sauté for 3 to 5 minutes, or until translucent.

Stir in the carrot, cumin, ginger, and salt. Cook, stirring, for about 1 minute. Add the squash and chicken broth. Bring to a boil; reduce the heat and simmer for about 20 minutes, or until the vegetables are tender.

Remove the pot from the heat. With an immersion blender or in a food processor (working in batches, if needed), purée the soup. Return the soup to the heat and stir in the coconut milk; season to taste with additional salt and pepper. Serve warm.

YAM AND BLACK BEAN CHILI

Chili is one of my family's favorites because it's easy, nourishing, and filling. The yams are a skin-soothing alternative to the typical tomato base. Because tomatoes, peppers, and other nightshade vegetables can trigger inflammation for many people with chronic skin issues, you won't find any of those ingredients in these recipes.

YIELD: about 6 servings

2 yams, peeled and cut into 1-inch (2.5 cm) cubes (about 3 cups, or 330 g)

1 tablespoon (15 ml) avocado oil

½ cup (80 g) chopped onion

2 cloves garlic, crushed or minced

1 pound (455 g) ground free-range turkey, grass-fed beef, or bison

2 cups (344 g) black beans, or 1 15-ounce (425 g) can, drained and rinsed

1 cup (235 ml) broth (chicken, beef, or vegetable)

1 teaspoon ground cumin

1 teaspoon turmeric

½ teaspoon dried oregano

½ teaspoon Himalayan salt or Celtic sea salt (or more to taste)

1 avocado, peeled, pitted, and cubed

¼ cup (4 g) minced fresh cilantro

1 tablespoon (15 ml) fresh lime juice

In a medium pot of boiling filtered water, cook the yams for 12 to 15 minutes, or until tender but not mushy. Drain and set aside.

Heat the avocado oil in a large soup pot over medium heat. Add the onion and garlic and sauté for a few minutes until translucent. Add the ground meat and cook, stirring, until browned.

Stir in the cooked yams, black beans, broth, cumin, turmeric, oregano, and salt. Cover and simmer for 5 minutes.

In a small bowl, gently combine the avocado, cilantro, and lime juice.

Serve the chili warm, topped with the avocado mixture.

BEANS AND GREENS SOUP

While meat can be a great source of iron, zinc, vitamin B12, and collagen, we don't need it every day. In fact, it's better for our environment and our health if we don't go overboard. This vegan recipe is so hearty, you'll forget it doesn't contain meat!

YIELD: about 6 servings

1 tablespoon (14 g) organic virgin coconut oil
1 cup (160 g) diced onion (yellow or white)
1 cup (130 g) sliced carrots
2 cloves garlic, minced
5 cups (1.2 L) broth of choice
3 cups (516 g) cooked black beans, or 2 15-ounce
   (425 g) cans, drained and rinsed

1 teaspoon dried oregano
3 cups (108 g) washed, chopped Swiss chard,
   or fresh organic spinach
1 teaspoon dulse (optional)
½ teaspoon Himalayan salt or Celtic sea salt
   (or more to taste)
Pepper

Heat the coconut oil in a large soup pot over medium heat. Add the onion, carrots, and garlic, and sauté until the onion is translucent.

Stir in the broth, black beans, and oregano; bring to a boil. Reduce the heat to medium-low and stir in the Swiss chard. Simmer for 10 to 15 minutes. Sprinkle with dulse (if using), and season to taste with salt and pepper. Serve warm.

BISON VEGGIE STEW

There's nothing like stew to warm and nourish the body. Compared to beef, buffalo meat is leaner, has a healthier balance of fats, and has higher amounts of iron and vitamin B12. Bison typically aren't given hormones or antiobiotics, so if you can't find it, go for grass-fed beef.

YIELD: about 6 servings

1 tablespoon (15 ml) avocado oil
1 pound (455 g) buffalo stew meat,
   or grass-fed beef
6 cups (1.4 L) Bone Broth (page 130)
1 medium onion, thinly diced
1 clove garlic, peeled
1 or 2 bay leaves

1 teaspoon Himalayan salt or
   Celtic sea salt (or more to taste)
½ teaspoon pepper
½ teaspoon paprika
Dash ground allspice, or ground cloves
3 large carrots, sliced
3 ribs celery, chopped
2 large parsnips, cubed

In a large soup pot over medium-high heat, heat the avocado oil. Add the meat and cook, stirring occasionally, until browned. Add the bone broth, onion, garlic, bay leaves, salt, pepper, paprika, and allspice. Cover and simmer for 1½ hours. Remove and discard the bay leaves and garlic clove. Add the carrots, celery, and parsnips. Cover and cook for 30 to 40 minutes. Serve warm.

SUMMER SOUPS

These soups, served chilled, are great on warm days or any time you're feeling overly warm.

WATERMELON GAZPACHO

This is a top pick for warm spring and summer days, when watermelon is in season and you can enjoy the skin-enhancing benefits of lycopenes and other nutrients in this pink fruit. For a creamier soup, blend in the almonds instead of using them as a garnish.

YIELD: 4 servings

2½ cups (375 g) seeded, cubed watermelon
1 cup (135 g) diced cucumber
½ cup (120 ml) filtered water
½ cup (8 g) loosely packed chopped fresh cilantro
⅓ cup (55 g) diced white onion
1 tablespoon (15 ml) fresh lime juice

1 teaspoon apple cider vinegar
¼ to ½ teaspoon grated fresh ginger
2 pinches Himalayan salt or Celtic sea salt (or more to taste)
½ cup (55 g) sliced raw almonds
Extra-virgin olive oil, for garnish

In a blender or food processor, place all ingredients *except* the almonds and olive oil. Quickly blend until smooth. Add additional salt to taste, and garnish each serving with ¼ cup (27.5 g) of almonds and a drizzle of olive oil.

RECIPE NOTE   Watermelon is an excellent source of the antioxidants lycopene, vitamin C, and beta-carotene. This juicy fruit is 92 percent water, meaning it's packed with hydration benefits.

CHILLED AVOCADO SOUP

This cool, refreshing soup's main ingredient is one of my all-time favorite skin-nourishing foods: avocado. Mixed with cilantro, lime juice, and ginger, this zesty bowl is sure to tickle your taste buds.

YIELD: about 8 servings

4 cups (946 ml) Chicken Bone Broth or
    Vegetable Broth (see variations, page 130)
3 ripe avocados, peeled and pitted
½ cup (17.5 g) fresh basil, or Italian parsley
½ cup (8 g) fresh cilantro
2 tablespoons (30 ml) fresh lime juice

2 teaspoons (10 ml) apple cider vinegar
1 teaspoon peeled, chopped fresh ginger
½ teaspoon Himalayan salt or Celtic sea salt
    (or more to taste)
Extra-virgin olive oil, for garnish
Pine nuts, for garnish

In a blender, combine the broth, avocados, basil, cilantro, lime juice, cider vinegar, ginger, and salt. Blend until smooth, but don't over-blend or the soup will heat up and become too thick. Refrigerate until cold.

To serve, garnish with a swirl of olive oil and a sprinkling of pine nuts.

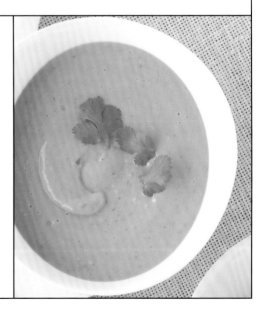

Fermented foods require a bit of prep time. *Please follow the instructions carefully.* Enjoy 1 to 2 serving per day of these probiotic-rich foods to support a healthy microbiome (a serving is about ½ cup or 70 g). Here are a few tips for making fermented foods:

- Do not use plastic or metal containers. Glass jars work great. I prefer those with swing-top lids, but Mason jars work well too. You can make larger batches in a slow cooker, but with larger batches the fermentation process takes longer.

- Sanitize all jars and utensils in boiling water or in the dishwasher. You don't want harmful bacteria growing with the healthy probiotics.

- Wash all vegetables well.

- Wash your hands well before and during preparation.

- Store fermented foods in a cool, dry place away from sunlight. I store mine in a dry cooler at a cool room temperature. I haven't seen it happen, but I've heard stories of glass containers shattering from the pressure of the fermentation process; I'd rather be safe and store them in a confined space.

- Label each batch with the name of the food, the date, and time it was made to help you keep track of passing time.

- The ideal temperature for fermentation is between 65°F and 75°F (18°C to 24°C), so on hot days, look for a cooler place.

- It can take up to two weeks to ferment vegetables; plan ahead so you have these available during your two-week program.

- While foods ferment, you may see bubbles, foam on top, or white scum. This is normal. You're growing probiotics, so that's a good sign!

- After foods are finished fermenting, keep them refrigerated. Fermented vegetables last a long time refrigerated. Even a year later, they are still safe to eat, though they will not contain as many beneficial microorganisms at that time. Use coconut yogurt within one week.

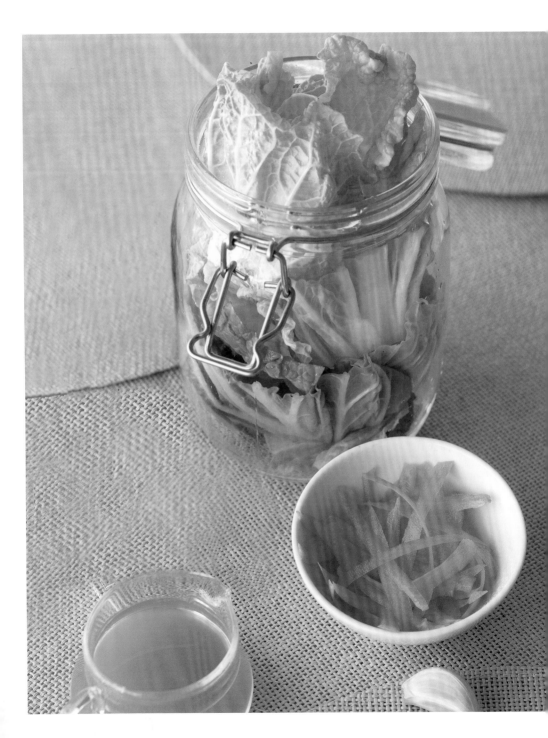

SAUERKRAUT

Sauerkraut takes some time to ferment, but you'll be able to enjoy it for months afterward. And you'll obtain the double benefit of a microbiome-enhancing fermented vegetable plus the cleansing benefits of cabbage (from the brassica family).

YIELD: about 8 cups (1.14 kg)

EQUIPMENT

2 small jars with lids
1 2-qt (2 L) jar or 2 1-qt (1 L) jars
Clean marbles or rocks

FOR SAUERKRAUT

1 head napa cabbage, or green cabbage
1 tablespoon (18 g) fine Himalayan salt
  or Celtic sea salt

FOR PASTE (OPTIONAL)

¼ cup (25 g) chopped scallions
¼ cup (27.5 g) grated carrot
2 tablespoons (20 g) chopped garlic
2 tablespoons (30 ml) apple cider vinegar
1 tablespoon (9 g) coconut palm sugar

Wash the food, jars, and equipment so you're working with a clean environment. Fill the small jars with clean marbles or rocks, and secure their lids.

To make the sauerkraut: Quarter the cabbage lengthwise, remove the cores, and then cut each quarter in half lengthwise. Thinly slice each section. Transfer to a large bowl.

Add the salt and massage the cabbage for about 5 minutes with your clean hands, or until coated and slightly wilted. Set aside.

If you want your sauerkraut simple (without spice), skip the paste and place the cabbage in the jars as instructed.

To make the paste (if using): In a medium bowl, mix together the scallions, carrot, garlic, cider vinegar, and coconut palm sugar. Add the paste to the cabbage and massage for 3 to 5 minutes.

Pack the cabbage into the large glass jars, packing it tightly with your fist or a spoon. Leave at least 1 inch (2.5 cm) of space at the top for the weighted jars to fit.

Place the weighted jars inside. If using Mason jars, cover the Mason jar and the inserted weighted jar with fabric and secure it with a rubber band. If using swing-top jars, secure the lid after inserting the weighted jar.

Let the cabbage sit in a covered container, such as a cooler, where it will get no sunlight. After 24 hours, the liquid should have risen above the cabbage (this helps prevent mold growth). If not, press the cabbage down and add brine (1 teaspoon fine Himalayan salt or Celtic sea salt plus 1 cup [235 ml] filtered water). Check this daily for the first few days.

Let ferment for 3 to 10 days (or longer). If you see any mold, skim it off, and make sure the cabbage is fully submerged. After 3 to 10 days, taste the sauerkraut; when it tastes good to you, remove from storage, cover the jar with its lid, and refrigerate. It should keep for 2 months or longer.

PICKLED BEETS WITH CUMIN AND GINGER

Here's another option packed with double benefits! This one's fermented and beet-centered, which offers nutritive and cleansing properties—not to mention the cumin and ginger, which make this recipe anti-inflammatory too.

YIELD: about 8 cups (1.8 kg)

5 to 6 medium beets, washed, peeled, and cut in
¼-inch (0.6 cm) slices
1 teaspoon cumin seeds, or coriander seeds
1-inch (2.5 cm) piece fresh ginger, peeled and
sliced into matchsticks

2 cups (475 ml) warm filtered water
1 tablespoon (15 g) fine Himalayan salt or
Celtic sea salt

Wash the food, jars (1 small jar with a lid, and 1 1-quart [946 ml] wide-mouth jar), and equipment so you're working with a clean environment. Fill the small jar with clean marbles or rocks, and secure the lid.

In a saucepan of boiling water, cook the beets for about 3 minutes. Remove from the heat, drain, and cool.

In the bottom of the wide-mouth jar, place the cumin seeds and ginger. Add the beets.

In a medium bowl, make the brine by combining the water and salt. Cover the beets with the brine, leaving about 1½ inches (3.5 cm) of headspace at the top of the jar. Place the small weighted jar on top of the beets, and cover both jars with a cloth, securing it with a rubber band. Place the jar on a small plate in case the fermenting liquid spills over. Ferment at room temperature, 65°F to 75°F (18°C to 24 °C), for 1 to 2 weeks.

CREAMY COCONUT YOGURT

Just because you're giving up dairy during the program doesn't mean you should miss out on the health benefits of yogurt. This coconut yogurt is naturally sweet and can be enjoyed as a thick beverage or a light yogurt.

YIELD: 1 pint (475 ml)

2 cups (475 ml) organic unsweetened coconut milk (homemade or purchased)

2 tablespoons (15 g) tapioca starch (tapioca flour)

4 probiotic capsules, or culture starter

2 tablespoons (18 g) coconut palm sugar

In a saucepan over medium heat, warm the coconut milk just until it starts to simmer. Transfer ½ cup (120 ml) to a small bowl and whisk in the tapioca starch. The mixture will thicken. Add this back to the saucepan and simmer for about 3 minutes, stirring constantly until thickened. Turn off the heat and cool the milk to 90°F to 100°F (32°C to 38°C).

Stir in the probiotics and coconut palm sugar. Pour the milk into a clean pint-size (475 ml) jar. Place the jar in a dry cooler at room temperature and let ferment for 12 to 24 hours. Then refrigerate for at least 6 hours to chill. Serve cold alone or with fresh berries or granola. Use within 1 week.

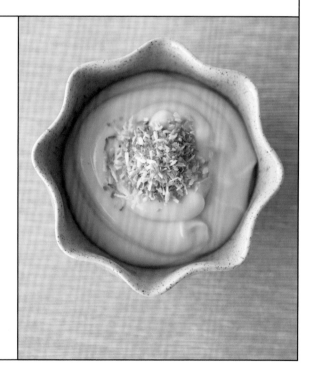

These recipes are some of my favorite skin-nourishing recipes for lunch or dinner. You won't find any of the foods to avoid here. Instead I've replaced them with the top foods for skin. These meals are balanced and nutritious, and I think you'll find them delicious!

BAKED GOLDEN CHICKEN WITH APPLES AND YAMS

Every time I visit home, my parents make the most amazing chicken dinners, and I've worked hard to come up with a recipe to match theirs! This version of my family's favorite is savory and sweet. And, I've added magical turmeric to make it golden. We enjoy it with steamed veggies and red rice (antioxidant-rich and with a nutty flavor). Be sure to pour the drippings on top!

YIELD: 4 to 6 servings

1 whole organic, free-range chicken
1 to 2 tablespoons (15 to 30 ml) avocado oil (depending on the size of the chicken)
2 large yams, unpeeled, sliced into large pieces
1 organic apple, unpeeled, cored, and sliced
1 tablespoon (1.7 g) chopped fresh rosemary
1 tablespoon (2.5 g) chopped fresh sage
½ teaspoon turmeric

½ teaspoon ground curcumin
½ teaspoon Himalayan salt or Celtic sea salt (or more to taste)
⅓ cup (78 ml) apple juice, or Bone Broth (page 130)
1 cup (190 g) organic red rice, or brown rice
2 cups (475 ml) filtered water

Preheat the oven to 350°F (180°C, or gas mark 4). Rinse the chicken and place it in a large baking dish. Rub it all over with avocado oil. Add the yams and the apples to the dish. Sprinkle with rosemary, sage, turmeric, curcumin, and salt; pour in the apple juice. Bake for about 1 hour, or until the chicken juices run clear.

While the chicken cooks, cook the rice in the water according to the package directions.

Serve the rice, chicken, yams, and apples together, with steamed greens, asparagus, or broccoli on the side, if desired.

RECIPE NOTE Reserve the chicken carcass and any leftover chicken meat to make Chicken Soup with Rice and Veggies (page 147).

QUINOA FRITTERS WITH PORK CHOPS

Growing up in the southern part of the United States, my family made pork chops often, so I've always appreciated this dish when well prepared. Many people fry pork chops to prevent over-drying the meat. But baking them as recommended here, with fruit and juice, keeps the pork moist and delicately delicious. Quinoa fritters are the perfect healthy addition to my spin on this traditional Southern meal.

YIELD: 2 servings

FOR PORK CHOPS

2 pastured pork chops, 3 to 4 ounces (85 to 115 g) each
Avocado oil, for the chops
1 organic red apple, sliced
⅓ cup (48 g) fresh blackberries, or frozen (optional)
⅓ cup (55 g) diced red onion
⅓ cup (78 ml) apple juice
2 cloves garlic, minced
½ teaspoon dried oregano
¼ teaspoon Himalayan salt or Celtic sea salt (or more to taste)

FOR FRITTERS

2 cups (370 g) cooked quinoa
½ cup (112 g) mashed cooked yams
½ cup (80 g) finely diced red onion
½ cup (48 g) organic almond flour
½ cup (40 g) unsweetened organic shredded coconut
1 clove garlic, pressed
½ teaspoon ground cumin
¼ teaspoon Himalayan salt or Celtic sea salt (or more to taste)
2 tablespoons (28 g) organic virgin coconut oil

To make the pork chops: Preheat the oven to 350°F (180°C, or gas mark 4). Rub the pork chops with avocado oil and place them in a baking dish. Top with the apple, blackberries, red onion, apple juice, garlic, oregano, and salt. Bake for 30 to 35 minutes, or until the chops reach an internal temperature of 145°F (63°C).

To make the fritters: In a large bowl, mix the quinoa, yams, red onion, almond flour, coconut, garlic, cumin, and salt. Form the mixture into patties, pressing to hold together.

In a large skillet over medium heat, melt the coconut oil. Add the patties (in batches if needed) and cook for 5 to 7 minutes per side until golden. Set aside and keep warm.

Serve the chops with a warm fritter and green salad or steamed vegetable, such as broccoli or asparagus, if desired.

OVEN-ROASTED SALMON WITH BELUGA LENTILS AND SALSA VERDE

This is one of my favorite recipes in the whole book. The combination of savory salmon, black lentils, and tangy salsa is sure to satisfy your palate—and you can relax, knowing every ingredient is nourishing your skin from within.

YIELD: 2 servings

FOR SALSA VERDE

1 cup (16 g) finely chopped fresh cilantro leaves
½ cup (30 g) finely chopped fresh Italian
    parsley leaves
2 tablespoons (20 g) minced red onion
4 cloves garlic, minced
¼ cup (60 ml) extra-virgin olive oil
1 tablespoon (11 g) Dijon mustard
2 teaspoons (10 ml) apple cider vinegar
3 pinches Himalayan salt or Celtic sea salt
    (or more to taste)

FOR LENTILS

½ cup (96 g) dried beluga (black) lentils,
    or green lentils
2 cups (475 ml) filtered water

FOR SALMON

2 wild salmon fillets, 6 ounces (170 g) each
1 tablespoon (15 ml) avocado oil, plus more
    for coating the salmon
¼ teaspoon Himalayan salt or Celtic sea salt
    (or more to taste)
Pepper
1 lemon, cut into 8 slices
2 cloves garlic, chopped

To make the salsa verde: In a medium bowl, mix all the ingredients well and set aside. The salsa can also be made in advance and refrigerated for up to 3 or 4 days.

To make the lentils: In a small pot over medium-high heat, combine the lentils and water. Bring to a boil and cook for 10 to 20 minutes, or until tender but not soggy. Strain, set aside, and cover.

To make the salmon: Preheat the oven to 375°F (190°C, or gas mark 5). Rub the salmon with a little avocado oil and season to taste with salt and pepper.

In a baking dish, layer the lemon slices on the bottom. Place the salmon on top of the lemon bed. Bake for 10 minutes, or until firm and cooked through.

In a medium saucepan over medium heat, stir together the garlic, 1 tablespoon avocado oil, and the cooked lentils. Sauté for 2 minutes until the garlic is aromatic.

To serve: Divide the lentils between 2 plates. Top each serving with a piece of salmon and a spoonful of salsa verde.

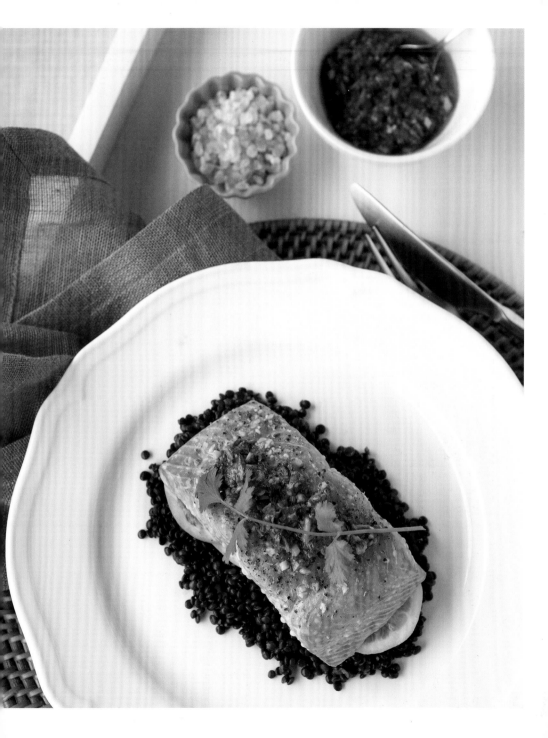

CHICKPEA GRIDDLECAKES WITH CILANTRO-COCONUT CHUTNEY

These griddlecakes are also great for breakfast served with some sliced avocado.

YIELD: 8 griddlecakes and about 2 cups (500 g) chutney

FOR CHUTNEY

1 cup (80 g) unsweetened organic shredded coconut

1 cup (16 g) fresh cilantro leaves

¾ cup (175 ml) filtered water

6 tablespoons (90 ml) fresh lime juice

2 tablespoons (12 g) chopped fresh mint leaves

1 tablespoon (15 ml) avocado oil

⅛ teaspoon Himalayan salt or Celtic sea salt (or more to taste)

FOR GRIDDLECAKES

2 cups (240 g) chickpea (garbanzo bean) flour

1½ teaspoons (3.75 g) ground cumin

½ teaspoon baking soda

½ teaspoon Himalayan salt or Celtic sea salt (or more to taste)

¼ cup (25 g) finely sliced scallions

¼ cup (4 g) finely chopped fresh cilantro

1 tablespoon (15 ml) fresh lemon juice

½ teaspoon minced fresh ginger, or ground ginger

1 cup (235 ml) filtered water

2 to 4 tablespoons (28 to 56 g) organic virgin coconut oil

To make the chutney: In a food processor, combine all the chutney ingredients and process until smooth. Set aside.

To make the griddlecakes: In a large bowl, mix the flour, cumin, baking soda, and salt. Stir in the scallions, cilantro, lemon juice, ginger, and enough water to form a pancake batter consistency.

In a griddle pan over medium heat, melt the coconut oil. Spoon or pour about ¼ cup (60 ml) of batter for each pancake onto the warm griddle. Cook for 3 to 5 minutes; flip and cook for 2 to 3 minutes more. Serve topped with the chutney.

Refrigerate any leftover chutney to enjoy with other meals.

CHICKEN SOUP WITH RICE AND VEGGIES

Ever since I read Maurice Sendak's *Chicken Soup with Rice* as a child, I've craved this warming, nourishing soup. At my house, after we consume a chicken dinner, I throw the leftover bones and meat in a slow cooker with water. The next day I'll whip up this recipe. If you prefer chicken noodle soup, add rice noodles instead of the rice, and allow enough time for the noodles to cook until tender but not mushy.

YIELD: about 8 servings

Leftover chicken meat and bones from Baked Golden Chicken with Apples and Yams (page 142)

Filtered water

4 large carrots, chopped

4 ribs celery, chopped

½ yellow or red onion, diced

3 cloves garlic, crushed

Himalayan salt or Celtic sea salt

Pepper

1 cup (200 g) cooked red rice, or brown rice

In a large soup pot over high heat, place the leftover chicken and bones. Add enough water to cover the chicken. Bring to a boil. Reduce the heat to low and simmer for 12 to 24 hours. Strain the broth to remove the bones, cartilage, and meat. Return the broth to the pot and place it over medium heat.

Add the carrots, celery, onion, and garlic. Season to taste with salt and pepper. Bring to a boil and then reduce the heat to low. Simmer for about 10 minutes, or until the carrots are tender. Stir in the rice and cook for 5 minutes more. Serve warm.

RECIPE NOTE If you don't have that leftover chicken carcass and meat in the fridge, you can still make this delicious soup. Instead of using leftover chicken meat and bones to make the broth, start with a whole 2- to 3-pound (1 to 1.5 kg) chicken and proceed according to the recipe. Or skip making the broth and start with 6 cups (1.4 L) of homemade Chicken Bone Broth (see variation, page 130); add 1½ cups (210 g) cooked, shredded chicken and continue with the recipe.

SALMON WITH LEMONGRASS GINGER BROTH AND WILTED GREENS

This recipe is completely different from my other salmon recipes but just as flavorful. Superfood salmon combined with lemongrass, ginger, cilantro, and kale make this meal satisfying and nourishing.

YIELD: 2 servings

FOR BROTH

2 cups (475 ml) Bone Broth (page 130)

1 stalk lemongrass, smashed, or 1 teaspoon lemongrass paste

2 tablespoons (12 g) peeled, chopped fresh ginger

FOR SALMON

2 pieces wild salmon, 4 to 6 ounces (115 to 170 g) each, or sustainably farmed salmon

Avocado oil, for coating the salmon

FOR CILANTRO SALSA GARNISH

2 tablespoons (2 g) chopped fresh cilantro

1 tablespoon (15 ml) extra-virgin olive oil

1 tablespoon (15 ml) fresh lime juice

1 clove garlic, minced

¼ teaspoon Himalayan salt or Celtic sea salt (or more to taste)

FOR SERVING

2 cups (134 g) kale

To make the broth: In a medium saucepan over medium heat, combine the bone broth, lemongrass, and ginger. Bring to a simmer and cook for 20 minutes. Strain out the lemongrass and ginger, reserving the liquid in the pan. Set aside. Just before serving, bring to a boil.

To make the salmon: Preheat the oven to 375°F (190°C, or gas mark 5). Rub the salmon with a little avocado oil and place it in a baking dish. While the broth simmers, bake the salmon for 10 to 15 minutes, or until cooked to your desired doneness.

To make the garnish: In a small bowl, mix all the ingredients; set aside.

To serve: Place 1 cup (30 g) of kale in each serving bowl. Ladle in ½ cup (120 ml) of broth. Top each bowl with 1 salmon fillet, and garnish with a spoonful of cilantro salsa. Serve warm.

PESTO SPAGHETTI SQUASH

Why overload on carb-heavy pasta when you can enjoy the nourishing benefits of spaghetti squash with tasty pesto? Like butternut, spaghetti squash is high in vitamins A and C and fiber. The difference is, once cooked, this squash can be separated with a fork into spaghetti-like strands, making it a perfect substitution for pasta.

YIELD: 2 to 4 servings, depending on the size of the squash

FOR SQUASH

1 large spaghetti squash, halved lengthwise, seeds and pulp removed
1 cup (235 ml) filtered water

FOR PESTO

2 cups (70 g) loosely packed fresh basil leaves
½ cup (67.5 g) pine nuts
½ cup (120 ml) extra-virgin olive oil
1 clove garlic
½ teaspoon Himalayan salt or Celtic sea salt (or more to taste)

To make the squash: Preheat the oven to 375°F (190°C, or gas mark 5). Place the squash halves, cut side up, in the baking dish, and pour the water into the bottom of the dish. Bake for about 40 minutes, or until easily pierced and shredded with a fork. When cool enough to handle, scrape the squash with a fork to create spaghetti-like strands; transfer strands to a large bowl.

To make the pesto: In a food processor combine the basil, pine nuts, olive oil, and garlic; process into a smooth paste. Season with salt.

Toss the pesto with the spaghetti squash and serve warm.

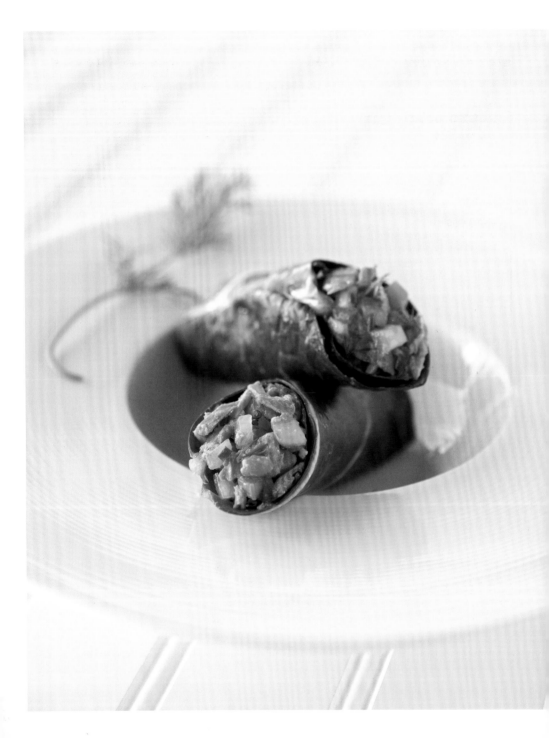

SALMON SALAD WRAPS

No mayonnaise or creamy dressing in this delectable salmon salad! And ditch the carbs and gluten when you use collard greens for the wraps. The crispness of the greens adds to this healthier sandwich's consistency, making it even tastier!

YIELD: 6 wraps

1 pound (455 g) wild salmon, cooked, chilled, deboned, and flaked; or canned wild salmon, drained
1 cup (135 g) peeled, diced cucumber
1 cup (120 g) thinly sliced celery
½ cup (80 g) diced red onion
1 tablespoon (15 ml) extra-virgin olive oil
1 tablespoon (15 ml) fresh lemon juice

1 tablespoon (4 g) fresh dill
1 tablespoon (4 g) chopped fresh parsley
1 tablespoon (3 g) chopped fresh chives
¼ teaspoon Himalayan salt or Celtic sea salt (or more to taste)
2 teaspoons (8 g) Dijon mustard
6 collard green leaves

In a large bowl mix the salmon, cucumber, celery, and red onion.

In a small bowl, whisk the olive oil, lemon juice, dill, parsley, chives, and salt. Add the dressing to the salmon mixture, and stir gently to combine.

Place ½ cup (about 60 g) of salmon salad on a collard green leaf and roll it up like a wrap. Repeat with the remaining ingredients.

COCONUT–RED LENTIL SOUP WITH CHICKPEA GRIDDLECAKES

This is a favorite among my vegan friends, and even meat-eaters will love the flavorful creamy soup and mouthwatering griddle-cakes. Enjoy any leftover chutney with other meals.

YIELD: about 8 servings

2 cups (384 g) dried red lentils

2 tablespoons (28 g) organic virgin coconut oil

½ cup (80 g) diced yellow onion, or red onion

1 clove garlic, minced or pressed

2 teaspoons (4 g) fennel powder

2 teaspoons (4 g) ground coriander

1 teaspoon minced fresh ginger, or ground ginger

1 teaspoon turmeric

1 teaspoon ground cumin

4 cups (946 ml) Vegetable Broth or Chicken Bone Broth (see variations, page 130)

1 teaspoon Himalayan salt or Celtic sea salt (or more to taste)

½ teaspoon pepper (or more to taste)

2 cups (475 ml) organic unsweetened coconut milk

4 cups (120 g) fresh organic baby spinach leaves, divided

1 batch Chickpea Griddlecakes (page 146)

If you have time, soak the lentils for 30 minutes to 3 hours before cooking. Rinse and drain the lentils until no more suds appear. In a large pot over medium heat, heat the coconut oil. Add the onion and garlic and sauté for about 3 minutes, or until the onion is translucent.

Stir in the fennel powder, coriander, ginger, turmeric, cumin, and lentils. Sauté for about 2 minutes.

Add the broth, salt, and pepper and bring to a boil. Reduce the heat to low. Cover and cook for 15 to 20 minutes. Stir in the coconut milk and cook for 15 minutes, or until the lentils are soft. Taste and adjust the seasonings if needed.

To serve: Place ½ cup (15 g) of spinach in each bowl and ladle the soup over it. Serve warm with griddlecakes.

THAI CHICKEN SALAD

Refreshing and satisfying, this chicken salad contains red cabbage, scallions, walnuts, and fresh herbs for an antioxidant boost. I include grains in some of the recipes for balance, but if you've gone grain free, skip the rice noodles.

YIELD: 8 servings

¼ cup (60 ml) extra-virgin olive oil

2 tablespoons (30 ml) fresh lime juice

¼ cup (4 g) chopped fresh cilantro

1 tablespoon (6 g) chopped fresh mint

1 teaspoon grated fresh ginger

½ teaspoon Himalayan salt or Celtic sea salt (or more to taste)

2 pounds (1 kg) cooked, shredded chicken breast, cooled

2½ cups (225 g) diced red cabbage

2 cups (352 g) cooked rice noodles, cooled

3 tablespoons (22.5 g) chopped walnuts

3 tablespoons (18 g) chopped scallions

8 large iceberg lettuce leaves, or butter lettuce, cabbage, or collard greens

In a small bowl whisk the olive oil, lime juice, cilantro, mint, ginger, and salt. Set aside.

In a large bowl, mix the chicken, red cabbage, rice noodles, walnuts, and scallions. Stir in the dressing and season with additional salt, if desired. Divide the salad among the lettuces leaves, wrap, and serve.

VARIATION   Instead of in a wrap, serve the chicken salad on a bed of greens.

These salads and other plant-based sides can be served with any of the main dishes or alone as a snack or a light meal. If you're enjoying these as the latter and the recipe doesn't contain nuts, seeds, or legumes, I recommend adding a serving of protein for a more balanced plate.

RAW "PASTA" SALAD

This is a refreshing way to serve zucchini and yellow squash, and it can make an excellent alternative to the traditional carb-heavy pasta salad. Using a spiralizer makes this quick and easy. My children love to help prepare this one, and I think it's fun to eat as well!

YIELD: 4 servings

2 medium zucchini, spiralized

2 medium yellow squash, spiralized

2 tablespoons (20 g) raw organic pumpkin seeds

2 tablespoons (30 ml) extra-virgin olive oil

1 tablespoon (2.5 g) chopped fresh basil

1 tablespoon (4 g) fresh dill

1 tablespoon (4 g) chopped fresh parsley

1 teaspoon apple cider vinegar

Himalayan salt or Celtic sea salt

Pepper

In a large bowl, combine the zucchini, squash, pumpkin seeds, olive oil, basil, dill, parsley, and cider vinegar. Mix together well and season to taste with salt and pepper. Refrigerate until cold and serve.

RECIPE NOTE If you don't have a spiralizer, use a mandoline or vegetable peeler to create spaghetti-like ribbons, or slice the vegetables very thin.

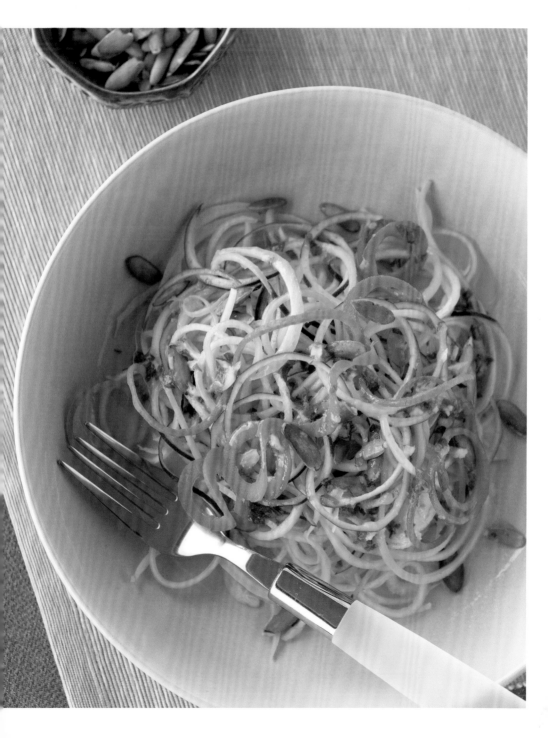

SIMPLE GREEN SALAD WITH TAHINI DRESSING

This green salad is easy to whip up, yet still deliciously skin nourishing. There are many variations you can make. Try other vegetables, or add fresh fruit. Leftover dressing can be used on other salads or as a vegetable dip.

YIELD: 4 to 6 servings as a side dish

FOR DRESSING

½ cup (120 ml) extra-virgin olive oil
¼ cup (60 g) tahini
2 tablespoons (30 ml) apple cider vinegar
2 tablespoons (30 ml) filtered water
1 tablespoon (15 ml) fresh lemon juice
1 teaspoon dried dill weed
1 teaspoon dried chives, or dried herb blend

FOR SALAD

8- to 10-ounce (225 to 280 g) package mixed greens, or 4 to 6 cups (220 to 330 g) lettuce of choice
1 cup (135 g) diced cucumber
1 cup (110 g) shredded carrot
1 cup (225 g) peeled, shredded beets

To make the dressing: In a small jar with a lid, combine the dressing ingredients. Cover tightly and shake well. Refrigerate while making the salad.

To make the salad: In a large bowl, combine all the salad ingredients. Toss the salad with enough dressing to coat the vegetables lightly before serving. Refrigerate any leftover dressing for another use.

BROCCOLINI SALAD

A cross between broccoli and kale, broccolini is almost akin to a young broccoli. Because this nutritious veggie is in the brassica family, it's a cleansing food and best served steamed. Serve this warm or cold with the tasty dressing.

YIELD: 2 servings

FOR SALAD

2 bunches broccolini, cut lengthwise into thin strips

½ cup (80 g) dried cherries (optional)

¼ cup (25 g) thinly sliced scallions

1 tablespoon to ¼ cup (12 to 48 g) cooked quinoa (optional for texture)

1 tablespoon (4 g) chopped fresh tarragon

FOR DRESSING

2 tablespoons (30 ml) extra-virgin olive oil

1 tablespoon (15 ml) fresh lemon juice

1 teaspoon filtered water

1 clove garlic, minced or pressed

1 tablespoon (8 g) sesame seeds

1 teaspoon grated fresh ginger

½ teaspoon ground cumin

½ teaspoon Himalayan salt or Celtic sea salt (or more to taste)

To make the salad: Steam the broccolini for 2 to 6 minutes until tender but still bright green. Remove from the steamer and place in cold water to stop the cooking. Removed, pat dry, and place in a large bowl.

Add the cherries (if using), scallions, quinoa (if using), and tarragon; toss to combine.

To make the dressing: In a small bowl, whisk the olive oil, lemon juice, water, garlic, sesame seeds, ginger, cumin, and salt. Pour as much dressing over the salad as you like, and toss to coat. Serve warm or cold.

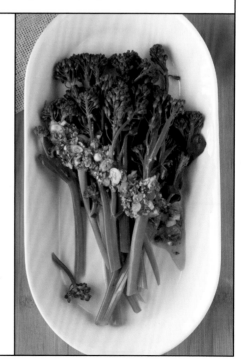

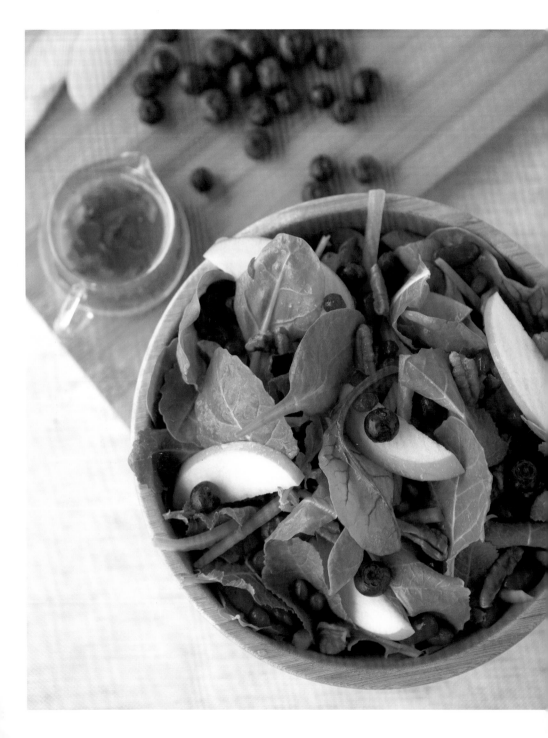

CRISP ANTIOXIDANT SALAD

The greens, carrots, blueberries, and pomegranate seeds fill this salad with vitamin C and the antioxidant family of carotenes, especially beta-carotene, lutein, and zeaxanthin. Human studies have shown carotenoid-rich diets can protect skin against sun damage by increasing its defense against UV light–mediated damage. In addition, walnuts are a nutrient-dense food and full of vitamin E and essential fatty acids for glowing skin.

YIELD: about 4 servings as a side dish

FOR SALAD

5-ounce (140 g) package power greens, baby kale, or salad mix

1 carrot, cut into thin matchsticks

½ cup (128 g) cooked kidney or red beans; or canned, rinsed and drained

½ organic Granny Smith apple, cut into thin wedges

½ cup (56 g) chopped raw pecans

½ cup (72.5 g) fresh organic blueberries

¼ cup (43.5 g) pomegranate seeds (optional)

FOR DRESSING

¼ cup (60 ml) extra-virgin olive oil

2 tablespoons (30 ml) apple cider vinegar

1 tablespoon (1 g) chopped fresh cilantro

1 tablespoon (2.5 g) chopped fresh basil

1 teaspoon dried oregano

1 teaspoon Dijon mustard

Himalayan salt or Celtic sea salt

Pepper

To make the salad: Toss all salad ingredients together in a large salad bowl.

To make the dressing: In a small bowl, whisk the olive oil, cider vinegar, cilantro, basil, oregano, and mustard. Season to taste with salt and pepper. When ready to serve, pour the dressing over the salad. Toss and enjoy.

ROASTED BRUSSELS SPROUTS AND CAULIFLOWER

If you love brussels sprouts, you'll love this recipe—and if you haven't tried baked brussels sprouts, you're in for a treat. Baking cauliflower and brussels sprouts (two of my favorite brassica veggies) makes them crisper and more flavorful than the soggy steamed version. The fresh thyme and lemon juice cut the bitter taste that makes some people averse to this vegetable family. Pomegranate seeds, when in season, make a terrific garnish.

YIELD: 4 servings

2 cups (176 g) brussels sprouts, halved
2 cups (200 g) chopped cauliflower florets (about 1 small head cauliflower)
2 to 3 tablespoons (30 to 45 ml) avocado oil
½ teaspoon Himalayan salt or Celtic sea salt (or more to taste)

3 tablespoons (33 g) pomegranate seeds (optional)
1 tablespoon (15 ml) fresh lemon juice
1 teaspoon chopped fresh thyme

Preheat the oven to 375°F (190°C, or gas mark 5); line a baking sheet with parchment paper.

In a large bowl, or on the baking sheet, mix the brussels sprouts, cauliflower, avocado oil, and salt. Spread the vegetables evenly on the sheet and roast for 20 minutes. When the veggies are soft but not mushy, remove from the oven and transfer to a large bowl.

Sprinkle on the pomegranate seeds (if using), lemon juice, and thyme. Toss to combine. Season with additional salt and avocado oil, if desired. Serve warm.

YUMMY GREENS

Don't feel you have to force down greens to abide by this diet. Take my word for it: Greens can be yummy! Whether you're already a fan or they're new to your diet, I think you'll love this simple greens recipe. Swiss chard is my favorite for this one.

YIELD: about 4 servings

2 tablespoons (30 ml) avocado oil
½ cup (80 g) diced yellow onion
2 cloves garlic, minced

6 cups (180 g) chopped fresh organic spinach, collard greens, kale, or Swiss chard
Himalayan salt or Celtic sea salt

In a large skillet over medium heat, heat the avocado oil. Add the onion and garlic and sauté for 2 to 3 minutes, until the onion is translucent. Slowly mix in the greens, stirring continuously until they are slightly wilted. Do not overcook. Season to taste with salt and serve.

REAL GREEN BEANS

You won't find canned green beans or mushroom soup in this recipe. Replace that green bean casserole at your family's next gathering with these fresh and flavorful veggies. Avoid overcooking this legume so the beans are not mushy or depleted of nutrients. The dressing ensures that this dish is anything but bland.

YIELD: about 6 servings

1 pound (455 g) green beans, trimmed
1 tablespoon (15 ml) extra-virgin olive oil
1 tablespoon (15 ml) fresh lemon juice
1 tablespoon (10 g) minced shallots
3 to 4 teaspoons (4 to 5 g) chopped fresh dill

1 teaspoon Dijon mustard
¼ teaspoon Himalayan salt or Celtic sea salt
  (or more to taste)
¼ teaspoon pepper

In a large saucepan (preferably one fitted with a steamer basket), bring about an inch (2.5 cm) of filtered water to a boil. Add the green beans; cover and cook for 5 to 7 minutes, until tender but still crisp.

In the meantime, in a large bowl, whisk the olive oil, lemon juice, shallots, dill, mustard, salt, and pepper. Add the green beans and toss to coat. Let stand for about 5 minutes to enhance the flavor before serving. Serve warm or cold.

LOW-CARB MASHED "POTATOES"

Instead of the typical mashed potatoes with butter and cream, enjoy the cleansing benefits of cauliflower and the same creamy texture with flavorful chives and garlic. Enjoy this recipe with garlic, but keep in mind a little goes a long way; it can quickly become overwhelming if you add too much.

YIELD: 4 servings

1 medium head cauliflower, cored and cut
  into small florets
2 ribs celery, chopped
½ cup (120 ml) organic unsweetened
  coconut milk

¼ cup (60 ml) extra-virgin olive oil
½ teaspoon Himalayan salt or Celtic sea salt
  (or more to taste)
¼ teaspoon minced garlic
2 tablespoons (6 g) chopped fresh chives

Steam or boil the cauliflower and celery until cooked, but not overdone. Drain well. With an immersion blender or in a food processor, purée the cooked cauliflower and celery with the coconut milk, olive oil, salt, and garlic. Blend until the mixture is the consistency of mashed potatoes. Garnish with additional olive oil and chives. Serve immediately.

QUINOA SALAD

When it comes to antioxidants in food, people often think of fruit and vegetables, but colorful grains and beans are also an excellent source. Red and black quinoa have higher amounts of polyphenols and antioxidant activity than regular quinoa. This salad calls not only for colorful quinoa and black beans but also some antioxidant-rich veggies, olives, herbs, and spices.

YIELD: 6 servings

1 cup (172 g) cooked black beans, or ½ cup (86 g) cooked black beans and ½ cup (120 g) cooked garbanzo beans

1 cup (135 g) diced cucumber

½ cup (50 g) chopped pitted green olives, or kalamata olives

4 red radishes, chopped

¼ cup (40 g) raw organic pumpkin seeds

3 cups (555 g) cooked and cooled quinoa, red, black, or tricolored

3 to 4 tablespoons (45 to 60 ml) extra-virgin olive oil

2 tablespoons (12 g) chopped fresh mint

2 tablespoons (8 g) chopped fresh parsley, or other fresh herb of choice

1 tablespoon (15 ml) fresh lemon juice

1 teaspoon ground cumin (optional)

1 clove garlic, minced or pressed

⅛ teaspoon Himalayan salt or Celtic sea salt (or more to taste)

Mixed greens, or spinach, for serving

In a large bowl, stir together the beans, cucumber, olives, radishes, and pumpkin seeds. Add the quinoa and stir to mix.

In a small bowl, whisk the olive oil, mint, parsley, lemon juice, cumin, garlic, and salt. Pour over the quinoa mix and toss to coat. Serve over a bed of greens.

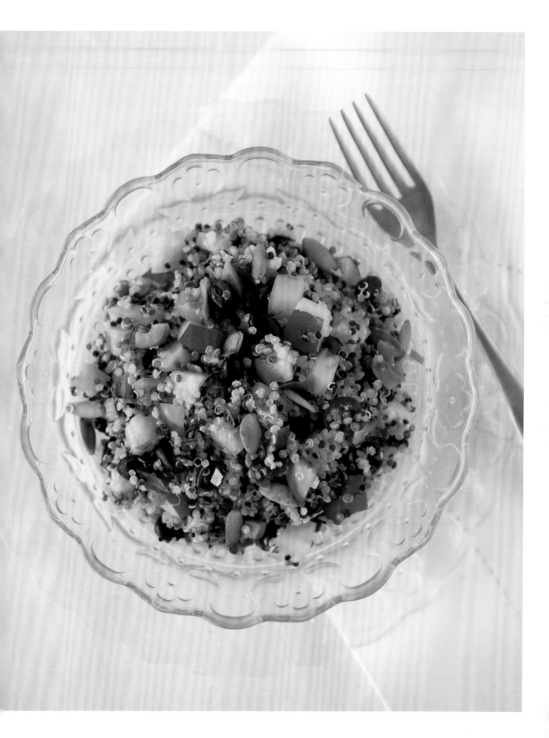

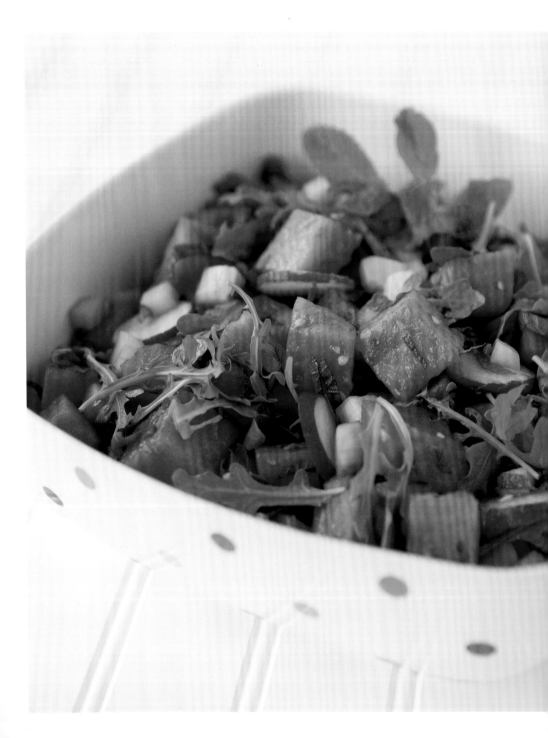

WATERMELON SALAD

Light and refreshing, this lycopene-rich watermelon salad also contains radishes, mint, cucumber, and lime—making it cleansing and replenishing. Because watermelon is seasonal and refreshing to the taste buds, it's best enjoyed during spring and summer.

YIELD: 10 servings

10 cups (1.5 kg) watermelon in 1-inch (2.5 cm) cubes, chilled
2 cups (270 g) diced cucumber
1 cup (116 g) sliced radishes
1 cup (96 g) minced fresh mint leaves
¼ cup (60 ml) extra-virgin olive oil
2 tablespoons (30 ml) fresh lime juice
¼ teaspoon Himalayan salt or Celtic sea salt (or more to taste)
4 cups (80 g) arugula

In a large bowl, mix the watermelon, cucumber, radishes, mint, olive oil, lime juice, and salt. Add the arugula and gently toss to combine. Serve chilled.

Enjoy these recipes between meals for easy and nutritious bites.

CRISP KALE CHIPS

These disappear quickly in my house. They're super simple to make, and are a great substitute for chips and other carb-heavy crunchy snacks. You can prepare them with oil and salt, or add a kick with cumin and turmeric.

YIELD: 4 to 8 servings

1 large head kale, about 4 cups (268 g), stalks removed, leaves cut into large pieces
2 tablespoons (28 g) melted organic virgin coconut oil

Himalayan salt or Celtic sea salt
Ground cumin
Turmeric or curry powder (optional)

Preheat the oven to 350°F (180°C, or gas mark 4). In a large bowl, coat the kale with coconut oil. Lay the kale pieces on a baking sheet in a single layer. Sprinkle to taste with salt, cumin, and turmeric or curry powder (if using). Bake for 5 to 10 minutes, or until the kale starts to turn crispy. Be careful not to burn. Remove from oven and serve.

BEAN DIP

It's always nice to have a yummy dip in the fridge when it's snack time. You can use a variety of cooked beans for this recipe and enjoy with sliced veggies, such as zucchini, carrots, and cucumbers. My favorite is garbanzo beans (chickpeas).

YIELD: about 2½ cups (600 g) dip

2 cups (364 g) cooked or canned beans of choice (white, garbanzo, black, or a mix)
¼ cup (60 g) tahini
¼ cup (60 ml) fresh lemon juice
¼ cup (60 ml) extra-virgin olive oil

1 clove garlic
1 teaspoon ground cumin
½ teaspoon Himalayan salt or Celtic sea salt (or more to taste)
2 to 4 tablespoons (30 to 60 ml) filtered water

In a food processor, combine the beans, tahini, lemon juice, olive oil, garlic, cumin, salt, and 2 tablespoons (30 ml) of water. Process until creamy and smooth. Thin with another 1 to 2 tablespoons (15 to 30 ml) of water, if you prefer. Refrigerate until ready to use. Use within 3 days.

GRAIN-FREE GRANOLA

This snack is also great for breakfast. You can add unsweetened dried fruit before baking, or fresh fruit afterward in a bowl with coconut yogurt or almond milk. You can also add the stevia to taste at the end.

YIELD: about 4 servings

2 tablespoons (28 g) organic virgin coconut oil
1 teaspoon pure vanilla extract
1 to 2 dashes powdered stevia (or more to taste)
1 cup (80 g) organic unsweetened organic coconut flakes (better to use than shredded)

½ cup (55 g) chopped pecans
½ cup (80 g) raw organic pumpkin seeds
½ teaspoon ground cinnamon
2 tablespoons (22 g) chia seeds

Preheat the oven to 350°F (180°C, or gas mark 4). Line a baking sheet with parchment paper and set aside. In small saucepan over low heat, melt the coconut oil. Turn off the heat and let the coconut oil cool for 1 minute. Stir in the vanilla and stevia powder.

In a medium bowl, mix the coconut, pecans, pumpkin seeds, and cinnamon. Stir in the coconut oil until the dry ingredients are well coated. Spread the granola on the prepared sheet and bake for 3 to 5 minutes, until just starting to brown. Remove from the oven and cool to room temperature.

RECIPE NOTE Feel free to substitute other nuts and seeds based on your preferences. You can also mix in no-sugar-added dried strawberries or raspberries.

SWEET QUINOA

Enjoy this sweet and healthy treat as a snack or for breakfast. In summer I sometimes skip the apple and toss in fresh berries after cooking.

YIELD: 2 servings

1 to 2 tablespoons (14 to 28 g) organic virgin coconut oil (less if the apple is juicy)
1 organic apple unpeeled, cut into small pieces
1 cup (185 g) cooked quinoa
¼ cup (35 g) dried pumpkin seeds (pepitas), or ½ cup (72.5 g) soaked almonds

2 tablespoons (10 g) unsweetened organic shredded coconut
¼ teaspoon ground cinnamon
¼ teaspoon ground ginger (optional)
Dash stevia powder

In a small saucepan over medium-low heat, melt the coconut oil. Add the apple and cook for about 5 minutes until tender. Stir in the quinoa, pumpkin seeds, coconut, cinnamon, ginger (if using), and stevia to taste. Cook until warmed through.

CHIA PUDDING

This bowl is raw, simple, and delicious. When chia seeds sit in liquid for 10 minutes, they absorb the fluid and transform into a tapioca-like consistency. If you don't care for tapioca's texture, blend the chia seeds with the other ingredients for a smoother consistency.

YIELD: 4 to 6 servings

½ cup (88 g) chia seeds

2 cups (475 ml) organic unsweetened almond milk, or unsweetened coconut milk

3 pitted dates, or stevia to taste

½ cup (68 g) cashews

½ teaspoon pure vanilla extract

½ teaspoon ground cinnamon

Pinch Himalayan salt or Celtic sea salt

¼ cup (20 g) unsweetened organic coconut flakes (optional)

¼ cup (36 g) fresh blueberries, or raspberries or pomegranate seeds (optional)

Place the chia seeds in a medium bowl. In a high-speed blender, combine the almond milk, dates, cashews, vanilla, cinnamon, and salt. Blend until creamy and smooth. Pour over the chia seeds and stir well to combine. Let sit for 10 to 15 minutes, or until the pudding thickens.

Serve at room temperature, or refrigerate and serve cold. Top with coconut and blueberries, if desired.

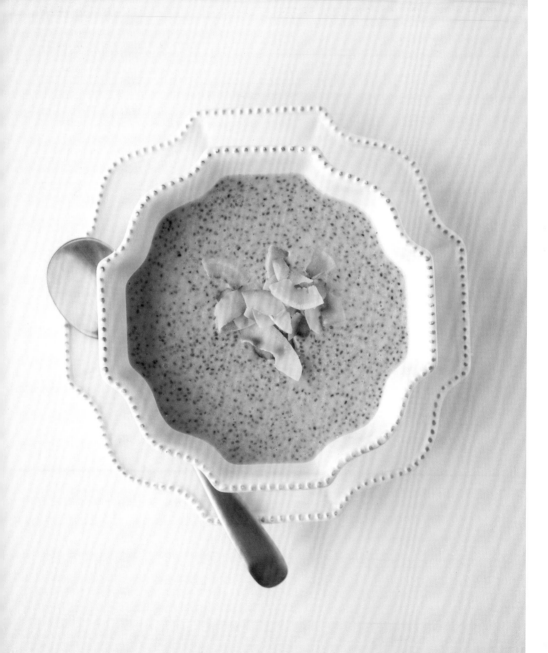

BAKED APPLE

Naturally sweet yet full of antioxidants and fiber, apples are a perfect sweet treat. Enjoy this as a snack or dessert. If serving as a dessert, add a spoonful of homemade Coconut Milk Whipped Cream (below).

YIELD: 4 servings

4 organic apples (any variety), cored

8 tablespoons (56 g) pecan pieces, or walnuts or cashews

2 teaspoons (4.6 g) ground cinnamon

2 teaspoons (3.6 g) ground ginger

2 teaspoons (10 ml) pure vanilla extract

4 dashes powdered stevia (optional)

Preheat the oven to 350°F (180°C, or gas mark 4). Place the apples in a baking dish. Cut a thin slice off the bottom, if needed, so they'll stand straight. Fill the center of each apple with 2 tablespoons (7 g) of pecans. Sprinkle each with ½ teaspoon cinnamon, ½ teaspoon ginger, and ½ teaspoon vanilla. Add a dash of stevia (if using). Bake for 45 minutes, or until tender.

COCONUT MILK WHIPPED CREAM

Whipped cream is the ultimate dessert topping, but when you try this coconut milk version, you may never go back to the traditional dairy version. Enjoy this on the peach cobbler, baked apples, or simply with a bowl of fresh fruit. Delish!

YIELD: 6 servings when served with Grain-Free Peach Cobbler (see right)

14-ounce (396 g) can coconut cream, or full-fat coconut milk

¼ cup (60 g) erythritol, or 1 dropperful of pure liquid stevia extract

½ teaspoon pure vanilla extract

Chill the can of coconut milk and a medium-size bowl in the refrigerator until cold. When cold, pour the coconut milk into the bowl; add the erythritol. With an electric mixer, whip the coconut milk for 10 to 15 minutes, or until fully whipped. Blend in the vanilla at the end.

Serve over Grain-Free Peach Cobbler (see right) or fresh fruit. Keep any leftovers chilled.

GRAIN-FREE PEACH COBBLER

Peach cobbler is another traditional Southern treat that is hard to give up, even during a two-week program. The good news is that this healthy version fits perfectly within your regimen. When in season, choose fresh organic peaches (preferably local), or use sliced frozen peaches from the grocery store.

YIELD: about 6 servings

FOR FRUIT FILLING

4 cups (680 g) sliced fresh organic peaches, or frozen and thawed
2 tablespoons (12 g) grated orange zest
2 tablespoons (30 ml) fresh orange juice

FOR TOPPING

½ cup (48 g) almond flour
½ cup (40 g) unsweetened organic coconut flakes
¼ cup (27.5 g) chopped pecans
¼ cup (27.5 g) sliced almonds
¼ cup (56 g) organic virgin coconut oil, melted, plus additional for greasing the baking dish
2 tablespoons (30 g) erythritol
¼ teaspoon ground cinnamon
¼ teaspoon ground ginger
Pinch Himalayan salt or Celtic sea salt (or more to taste)

Preheat the oven to 350°F (180°C, or gas mark 4). Grease an 8-inch (20 cm) round baking dish (or similar size) with coconut oil.

To make the filling: In a large bowl, mix the peaches, orange zest, and orange juice. Pour into the baking dish.

To make the topping: In a medium bowl, combine the flour, coconut, pecans, almonds, coconut oil, erythritol, cinnamon, ginger, and salt until crumbly. Scatter evenly over the fruit filling.

Bake for 40 to 50 minutes, until the fruit is bubbly. Serve warm with Coconut Milk Whipped Cream (see left).

CHAPTER 9

DIY Skin Care

In this chapter you will find simple DIY skin care recipes you can whip up at home and use during the two-week program.

Everything here is simple to prepare and use and includes reasonably priced, easy-to-find ingredients. Chances are you already have them in your kitchen.

The simplicity of these recipes mirrors the spirit of this book—if an ingredient is not good for you to eat, you shouldn't put it on your skin. As we now know, the whole body is connected, and what we put in and on our skin is reflected in our appearance.

All ingredients in these DIY recipes have the ability to help cleanse, balance, and nourish skin—naturally.

FIVE NATURAL INGREDIENTS FOR YOUR SKIN FROM YOUR KITCHEN

We've covered some of these items in chapter 4. Here's a quick refresher, with information on why they're perfect when it comes to DIY skin care.

1. Avocado is hydrating and nourishing, with naturally occurring vitamins A and E—it's great for masks.

2. Honey is healing, hydrating, clarifying, anti-inflammatory, antimicrobial, and pH balancing. It's great in skin cleansers, masks, and exfoliants. Remember to use raw (unpasteurized) honey; you don't want to kill this ingredient's beneficial bacteria.

3. Oats have moisturizing, anti-inflammatory, and healing properties. They're perfect in skin cleansers and masks.

4. Yogurt contains nutrients, enzymes, and active cultures that help reduce inflammation and balance skin's pH for a healthy skin microbiome. Use it alone as a skin soother or to make skin cleansers and masks.

5. Papaya contains the natural enzyme papain, which helps exfoliate skin, leaving it smooth and soft. It's full of antiaging benefits, so it's good for more mature skin as well. Greener (unripe) papayas have higher amounts of papain; opt for these to get the best exfoliation. If you have sensitive skin, use ripe papayas, which are less likely to trigger an inflammatory reaction.

TOP FOUR OILS
FOR DIY SKIN CARE

Nourish skin with naturally occurring vitamins E and A, as well as other important nutrients from these oils that help hydrate, clear, and rejuvenate it.

1. Coconut oil works well to remove makeup and surface buildup, and it possesses antimicrobial properties. The key to using coconut oil on any skin type—especially acne-prone Olivia-types (see pages 25–26)—is using a pure, extra-virgin source. Another bonus: Coconut oil does not become rancid as easily as some other oils, so it stays fresher longer.

2. Sunflower seed oil can help soothe and calm skin. Because it is thinner than some other oils, it works well in combination to make other oils easier to apply.

3. Sweet almond oil is a light, mildly scented oil that's gentle on skin and easily absorbed, making it a perfect DIY skin care ingredient.

4. Avocado oil is highly absorptive and great for dry or mature Sage-types (see pages 28–30). In addition to its hydrating qualities, its high antioxidant levels help heal and protect skin.

FIVE PLANT-BASED
SKIN SOOTHERS

The following ingredients naturally, brighten, balance, soothe, and cleanse skin.

1. Aloe vera gel has antimicrobial, anti-inflammatory, and healing properties, and it penetrates skin easily to provide nourishment. It's terrific for soothing skin overexposed to the sun, as well as for treating minor cuts and scrapes, eczema, and acne. The aloe you find in most stores contains preservatives, fillers, and artificial ingredients. Look for pure aloe at your local health food store; or buy an aloe plant, simply slice open a leaf, and extract and save the gel.

2. Black tea, made with loose-leaf tea or a tea bag, can help reduce redness and puffiness, as well as protect skin from the sun. Cool it in the refrigerator for use in DIY skin care.

3. White and green teas have anti-inflammatory, brightening, evening, cleansing, and hydrating properties. These are perfect ingredients for toners and masks, and the wide range of perks means they're helpful for most skin types. Due to antiaging compounds, they're ideal for mature Sage-types (see pages 28–30) as well. Follow the package instructions to make the teas, and cool them for use in DIY skin care.

4. Turmeric, with its anti-inflammatory and soothing properties, is great for Heath- and Emmett-types (see pages 26–28). Because of its anti-microbial, pore-cleansing, and sebum-balancing effects, it's perfect for Olivia-types (see pages 25–26)

as well. With its antioxidant properties and skin-evening benefits, Amber- and Sage-types (see pages 23–25 or 28–30) also benefit from skin care containing this powerful root. Avoid using it straight because its bright yellow color can stain skin.

5. Ginseng can help de-stress, rejuvenate, brighten, and balance skin, making it an ideal choice for Amber- and mature Sage-types (see pages 23–25 or 28–30). Its antioxidant, anti-inflammatory, and healing benefits offer relief for Olivia- and Heath-types (see pages 25–27) too.

TOP FOUR ESSENTIAL OILS FOR DIY SKIN CARE

As we discussed in chapter 4, the following four essential oils offer a good starting point for incorporation into your everyday skin care. Here are some specific benefits for your skin.

1. Tea tree essential oil has antimicrobial and anti-inflammatory properties and may help reduce acne breakouts for Olivia-types (see pages 25–26) with mild to moderate acne. Also known to help soothe seborrheic dermatitis and heal wounds, tea tree oil can benefit Emmett-types (see pages 27–28). Use tree oil essential oil diluted; the undiluted variety can burn and irritate skin when applied directly.

2. Ylang-ylang flower oil helps balance sebum levels for both overly dry and overly oily complexions. It also has a soothing and smoothing effect, and makes a great addition to DIY skin care for all skin types.

3. Clary sage contains natural antimicrobial agents, so it can be helpful in addressing wounds and skin infections.

4. Lavender has antimicrobial, anti-inflammatory, and immune-boosting effects. These benefits, plus pain-reducing and wound-healing properties, make lavender one of my favorite essential oils in skin care.

TIPS FOR DIY SKIN CARE

The DIY skin care recipes in this chapter are designed as part of my two-week program. For long-term daily skin care after the two-week program, I suggest using a high-quality natural skin care line, such as The Spa Dr.'s Daily Essentials.

▸ It's essential to use these DIY skin care recipes when they're fresh and refrigerated. Make a fresh batch every three days, and throw out any unused portions unless the recipe indicates otherwise. Some ingredients can grow bacteria and mold quickly, while other natural ingredients have antioxidant and antimicrobial properties that help keep the formula fresh. Caution: Just because something looks and smells okay doesn't mean harmful microorganisms aren't growing there.

▸ Natural ingredients can cause reactions and skin irritation in some people. If you know you react to any of the ingredients when you eat them, do not put them on your face.

▸ Even if you're not allergic to the product when you consume it, to be safe, do a patch test by applying it on the inside of your wrist before doing so anywhere else. For the next few hours, watch for any redness, swelling, or irritation to make sure you don't have a reaction. If you do, avoid the product.

▸ Use only distilled water for skin care, because it is free of contaminants. Non-distilled water makes products more likely to grow mold and bacteria.

▸ When you make a batch of product, store it in a jar or tightly sealed glass container in the refrigerator to preserve its freshness.

▸ Use products containing citrus juice and oils only at night; direct sun exposure after using citrus on the skin can increase your risk of sunburn, irritation, and hyperpigmentation.

▸ Products should feel smooth, not gritty. Avoid physical abrasion to the skin—we don't want to damage its texture or harm its microbiome.

These cleansers will not remove makeup unless they contain oils.

COCONUT MILK AND GRAPE JUICE CLEANSER

The hydrating effects of coconut milk and almond oil make this cleanser great for dry skin types, such as Emmett- and Sage-types (see pages 27–30). The antioxidant-rich grape juice makes it beneficial for dry Sage-types as well.

YIELD: 1 or 2 applications

1 tablespoon (15 ml) organic unsweetened coconut milk

2 teaspoons (10 ml) red or black grape juice
1 teaspoon sweet almond oil

In a small bowl, whisk together the coconut milk, grape juice, and almond oil. Gently massage over your face for a few minutes. Remove with a warm, wet washcloth.

If not using right away, re-whisk before applying, as the ingredients may separate.

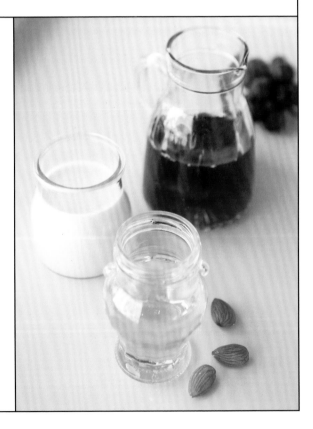

CHAMOMILE OAT CLEANSER

Great for Heath- and Emmett-types (see pages 26–28) because of its anti-inflammatory and skin-soothing benefits, even for sensitive skin.

YIELD: 4 or 5 applications

¼ cup (30 g) organic oats ground into a flour, or oat flour

1 organic chamomile tea bag
¾ cup (175 ml) hot distilled water

In a food processor, grind the oats into a fine (not gritty) powder; transfer to a medium bowl. In a mug, steep the chamomile tea in hot water for at least 3 to 5 minutes. Cool to room temperature.

Stir enough tea into the oat flour to make a paste. Wet your face with warm water and gently massage the cleanser over your face, avoiding the eye area. Rinse with warm water. Use within 2 days.

Alternatively, refrigerate the tea and flour separately, combining the ingredients when needed. Use the ingredients within 5 days.

EVENING AVOCADO AND LIME CLEANSER

Another great cleanser for drier skin—the oils in avocado cleanse, replenish, and moisturize skin, and the lime acts as a natural astringent. Use this cleanser only at night because direct sun exposure after using citrus on the skin can cause sun sensitivity.

YIELD: 6 or 7 applications

½ organic avocado
2 tablespoons (8 g) chopped fresh kale

½ teaspoon fresh lime juice

In blender or food processor, purée the avocado and kale. Add the lime juice and pulse to combine. Gently massage the mixture over your face for 3 minutes. Rinse with warm water. Lightly pat your face dry with a clean towel.

The lime juice helps keep this cleanser fresh for a few extra days, but use within 7 days.

ORGANIC HONEY AND TEA TREE CLEANSER

The antimicrobial and sebum-balancing effects of the honey and tea tree essential oil in this cleanser are great for Olivia-types (see pages 25–26).

YIELD: 3 to 5 applications

3 tablespoons (60 g) organic raw honey

2 drops pure tea tree essential oil

In a food processor, or by hand, vigorously mix the honey and tea tree oil. If the honey is too thick to blend, warm it slightly in a small saucepan over low heat. Remove it from the heat when it's just warm enough to become liquid. Do not boil. Mix in the tea tree oil and cool to room temperature before applying.

Lather the cleanser over your face, and gently massage it into your skin with your fingertips for 3 to 6 minutes. Gently tap skin, and then rinse with warm water.

ORGANIC APPLE, ALMOND OIL, AND YOGURT CLEANSER

The natural enzymes from the apple's malic acid and the lactic acid from the yogurt make this cleanser a good choice for Olivia- and Sage-types (see pages 25–26 or 28–30), and the almond oil helps balance sebum. This product cleanses without dehydrating.

YIELD: 7 or more applications

½ organic apple
¼ cup (60 g) unsweetened natural yogurt

1 tablespoon (15 ml) sweet almond oil

In a blender, process the apple to a pulp. Add the yogurt and almond oil; pulse to combine. Gently massage the blend over your face for a few minutes. Rinse with warm water. Refrigerate any unused cleanser.

The malic and lactic acids help keep this formula fresh for a few extra days, but use it within 7 days.

ORGANIC KIWI CLEANSING MILK

The natural enzymes in kiwi and yogurt make this is another good selection for Olivia-types (see pages 25–26). In addition, kiwi's vitamin C and alpha-hydroxyl acids support a glowing complexion for Sage-types (see pages 28–30).

YIELD: 3 or 4 applications

1 organic kiwi, peeled
2 tablespoons (30 g) organic plain yogurt

1 tablespoon (15 ml) sunflower seed oil

In a blender, combine the kiwi, yogurt, and sunflower oil. Mix thoroughly. Gently massage over your face for a few minutes and then rinse with warm water.

FACE TONERS

Toners are a second step to clean skin further and balance its pH after rinsing with water. As you'll see in chapter 10, I don't generally recommend commercial toners on a daily basis for most skin types unless they're needed to rebalance skin after cleansing. For the two-week program, I recommend the following DIY toners. In addition to cleaning and balancing, these recipes contain important nutrients and properties to enhance skin health.

MANGO JUICE TONER

Mango—great for Olivia skin types (see pages 25–26)—cleans and rejuvenates skin, keeping it soft and supple.

YIELD: 5 or 6 applications

½ small organic mango

In a blender, blend the mango to a juice; strain through a fine-mesh strainer to collect the juice. Transfer to a storage container and refrigerate. Pat onto your face with your fingertips, or saturate a cotton pad and wipe over your face. Keep any unused portions refrigerated; use within 3 days

BRIGHTENING RICE WATER TONER

The rice water in this skin toner is perfect for sensitive or inflamed Heath- and Emmett-types (see pages 26–28), but without the optional apple cider vinegar. For Amber-, Oliva-, and Sage-types (see pages 23–26 and 28–30), this toner, with the apple cider vinegar, helps brighten and even skin tone.

YIELD: about 8 applications

½ cup (50 g) cooked organic brown rice
½ cup (120 ml) warm distilled water

3 tablespoons (45 ml) apple cider vinegar (optional)

In a medium bowl, combine the rice with enough water to cover it. Stir and set aside for 10 minutes, or until the water turns cloudy. Drain the rice and reserve the water. Pour the water into a container, add the vinegar (if using), and refrigerate for about 30 minutes, or until cool but not cold. With your fingertips, pat onto your face, or spritz it on. You can also apply this to your chest, trunk, arms, and legs.

Keep any unused toner refrigerated and use within 3 days to avoid contamination.

GINSENG TONER

Ginseng helps rejuvenate, brighten, and balance skin, making it an ideal choice for Amber- and mature Sage-types (see pages 23–25 and 28–30). Its antioxidant, anti-inflammatory, and healing benefits can help Olivia- and Heath-types too (see pages 25–27).

YIELD: about 8 applications

1 ginseng tea bag (available at health food stores)

½ cup (235 ml) hot distilled water

Steep the ginseng tea bag in the hot water according to the package directions. Cool to room temperature, and then pat onto your face with your fingertips; or saturate a cotton pad and wipe over your face. Refrigerate for up to 1 week.

TEA TONER

Tea toner is perfect for hyperpigmented Amber- and mature Sage-types (see pages 23–25 and 28–30), as it helps naturally lighten and even complexions. Studies have shown that components in green tea reverse sun aging and improve pigmentation. It also has anti-inflammatory effects, which, in addition to the sebum-balancing effects of ylang-ylang, can also be helpful for Olivia-types (see pages 25–26).

YIELD: 2 or 3 applications

2 tablespoons (30 ml) steeped green, white, or black tea, made with distilled water, cooled

1 teaspoon sweet almond oil
2 drops ylang-ylang essential oil

With a hand mixer or in a blender, mix the green tea, sweet almond oil, and ylang-ylang oil. Pat onto your face with your fingertips.

ALOE-ROSE TONER

This toner is excellent for Heath- and Emmett-types (see pages 26–28). The natural astringent properties are gently vasoconstricting, but it's still nourishing, so it may decrease the appearance of redness and dilated capillaries without starving them of nourishment. Because the ingredients also have firming properties, this toner can be great for Sage-types too (see pages 28–30).

YIELD: 4 or 5 applications

3 tablespoons (45 ml) aloe vera gel

1 tablespoon (15 ml) rose water

In a small bowl, mix the aloe gel and rose water. Pat onto your face with your fingertips. Use within 3 days.

FACE EXFOLIANTS

Exfoliation helps remove dead skin from the surface to reveal glowing and vibrant skin. It's important not to over exfoliate because it can scratch and inflame your skin, as well as damage your skin's microbiome. Avoid abrasive mechanical and chemical exfoliants; instead use these DIY exfoliant recipes, ensuring the finished texture is smooth, not gritty.

If you're a Heath- or Emmett-type (see pages 26–28), exfoliation may be too irritating for sensitive or inflamed skin. If the skin on your face is dry but not inflamed, some exfoliators will be great for you to use. Amber, Olivia, and Sage skin types (see pages 23–30) will love the following exfoliant recipes. You can use these every three to seven days during the two-week program, and afterward if you choose.

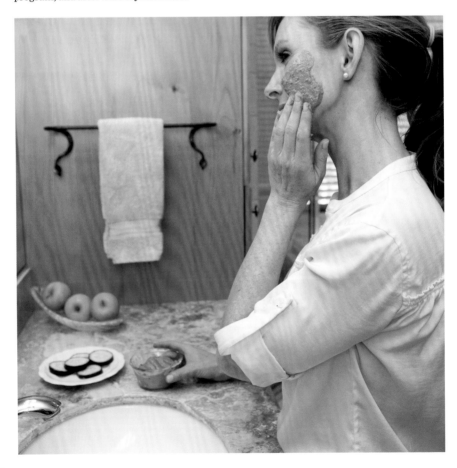

OATS AND OIL EXFOLIANT

This natural combination of ingredients gently exfoliates dead and dulling skin cells and brightens and reduces redness and discoloration to reveal fresh, bright, glowing skin. Please note that for some acne-prone skin types, the only oil they can tolerate (that doesn't trigger breakouts) is jojoba oil, but sweet almond oil is great for most people.

YIELD: 4 applications

½ cup (60 g) organic oats ground into a flour, or oat flour

1 tablespoon (15 ml) jojoba oil (for acne prone skin) or sweet almond oil (for dry skin)

In a small bowl, blend the oat flour and oil. Gently apply to damp skin using circular motions for 2 to 3 minutes. Rinse with warm water.

ORGANIC STRAWBERRY AND ALMOND EXFOLIANT

Strawberries naturally brighten skin and are rich in vitamin C; the almonds act as a natural and effective exfoliant. Ideal for Amber and Sage skin types (see pages 23–25 and 28–30), the antioxidants in this exfoliant reduce free radical- and inflammation-induced signs of aging and pigmentation.

YIELD: 3 applications

4 large organic strawberries

6 almonds ground to a smooth flour, or 1 tablespoon (6 g) almond flour

In a small bowl, mash or purée the strawberries to a pulp. Stir in the almond flour. Gently massage the mixture onto damp skin using circular motions for 2 to 5 minutes. Rinse with cool water.

Keep any unused portions refrigerated and use within 3 days.

PAPAYA SKIN EXFOLIANT

Papaya skins contain the natural enzyme papain, which acts as the exfoliant. This recipe is great for Amber-types as well as Olivia- and Sage-types (see pages 23–26 and 28–30). It may be too irritating for Heath- and Emmett-types (see pages 26–28).

YIELD: 1 application

Skin of 1 ripe papaya

Gently massage the inside of the papaya skin over your face for 2 to 3 minutes. Rinse with cool water.

POMEGRANATE AND VITAMIN E EXFOLIANT

This exfoliant is ideal for Amber and Sage skin types (see pages 23–25 and 28–30) because of its high antioxidant level. Pomegranate, honey, and vitamin E provide a whole host of essential skin-rejuvenating benefits.

YIELD: 4 applications

½ cup (87 g) pomegranate seeds (arils)
1 teaspoon organic raw honey

1 vitamin E liquid capsule (non-GMO)

In a blender, process the pomegranate seeds until smooth. Add the honey. Pierce the vitamin E capsule to release the liquid into the blender. Blend thoroughly. Gently massage over your face for 2 to 5 minutes. Rinse with warm water and a washcloth.

BROWN SUGAR AND CRANBERRY JUICE EXFOLIANT

Brown sugar contains glycolic acid and works as a great natural exfoliant. Once dissolved in cranberry juice, the sugar will be smooth and nonabrasive. If you don't have cranberry juice on hand, use pomegranate, grape, or pineapple juice instead.

This exfoliant is best for Olivia-types (see pages 25–26) when you do not have active inflamed acne. Do not use this exfoliant if you are a Heath- or Emmett-type (see pages 26–28), or have otherwise inflamed skin, because it may be irritating.

YIELD: 1 application

1 tablespoon (15 g) organic brown sugar

½ teaspoon cranberry juice, or aloe gel

In a small bowl, completely dissolve the brown sugar in the cranberry juice. Apply to your face and *gently* massage for 2 to 5 minutes. Rinse with warm water and a washcloth. Use only once per week.

Masks are my favorite part of DIY skin care, and there are so many natural options that can rebalance, hydrate, and nourish. You can enjoy masks daily or weekly during the two-week program, and beyond.

OAT, GREEN TEA, AND YOGURT FACE MASK

This combination is fantastic for sensitive or inflamed Heath- and Emmett-types (see pages 26–28) because of the anti-inflammatory and hydrating properties. The oats also help absorb excess oil, and the balancing effects of yogurt and green tea make it great for acne-prone Olivia-types (see pages 25–26). This mask doesn't have the photosensitivity issues of the Evening Papaya Mask (page 188), so you can use it year-round, any time of day.

YIELD: 3 or 4 applications

¼ cup (30 g) oat flour

2 tablespoons (30 g) plain organic yogurt

1 tablespoon (15 ml) brewed green tea, cooled

In a small bowl, mix the flour, yogurt, and green tea. Apply evenly to your face. Leave it on for 10 to 20 minutes; rinse with warm water.

TURMERIC-CHICKPEA FACE MASK

The three Cs in this mask—chickpeas, cucumber, and coconut—are soothing and healing for skin. Turmeric is ideal for its brightening effects for Amber and Sage skin types (see pages 23–25 and 28–30).

YIELD: 2 applications

2 tablespoons (15 g) chickpea flour

1 teaspoon cucumber juice

½ teaspoon organic unsweetened coconut milk

¼ teaspoon turmeric

In a small bowl, mix the flour, cucumber juice, coconut milk, and turmeric to form a paste. Add more flour if the paste is too thin. Apply the mask evenly to your face. Leave it on for about 15 minutes, but not until the paste dries. Rinse with warm water.

STRAWBERRY YOGURT FACE MASK

Brighten dull skin with this rejuvenating mask. Strawberries are rich in vitamin C and other antioxidants that offer skin brightening, lightening, and antiaging benefits for Amber- and Sage-types (see pages 23–25 and 28–30). They're good for oily and acne-prone Olivia skin (see pages 25–26) as well, as they help remove excess sebum. You're already aware of honey and yogurt's balancing and nourishing properties. If you are an Olivia-type, add clay for sebum-balancing effects. Note: If you have an allergy to berries, use ½ cup (75 g) cubed watermelon here instead.

YIELD: 4 applications

3 large organic strawberries, stemmed and roughly chopped

1 tablespoon (15 g) organic plain yogurt

1 tablespoon (20 g) organic raw honey

1 tablespoon (7.6 g) French green clay or bentonite clay (optional; for oily/acne skin types)

In a small bowl, thoroughly mash the strawberries with a fork, or purée them in a food processor. Add the yogurt, honey, and clay (if using); blend well. Apply the mask evenly to the skin. Leave it on for 10 to 20 minutes; rinse with warm water.

Keep refrigerated in a covered container, and use within 3 days of making. If you use clay, use the mask soon—it grows mold quickly.

EVENING PAPAYA MASK

Papaya is rich in vitamins A, C, and E and has antioxidant properties that help rejuvenate skin. Alpha hydroxy acids (AHAs) and papain help exfoliate. This mask is beneficial in treating acne and dark spots.

Use this mask only at night because, like citrus, AHAs can cause photosensitivity. If you have hyperpigmentation, this could make it worse if you go into the sun within 12 hours of use. Also be sure to use a mineral sunblock.

YIELD: 2 applications

1 tablespoon (14 g) ripe papaya flesh
1 tablespoon (15 g) organic plain yogurt (cow's milk or coconut milk)

1 teaspoon oatmeal

In a blender or food processor, process the papaya, yogurt, and oatmeal until smooth. Apply to your clean, dry face. Leave it on for 10 minutes, and rinse with warm water. Rinse your face again with cool water, and pat dry.

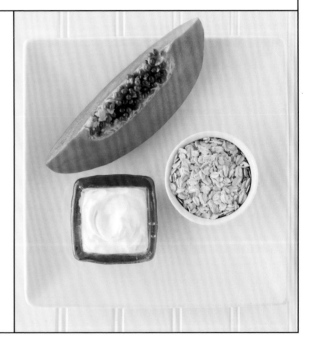

NATURAL BEAUTY FACE MASK (AND SMOOTHIE)

Rich in antioxidants with anti-inflammatory and nourishing benefits, this is great for all skin types and mild inflammation—but not for skin with open wounds or moderate to severe eczema, acne breakouts, or other eruptions. This recipe also doubles as a delicious smoothie (see below). If you want to save the remaining mask for your face rather than make a smoothie, it will keep refrigerated for 3 days.

YIELD: 1 mask treatment and 1 smoothie (see below)

¼ cup (36 g) raw almonds soaked in distilled water overnight, drained
¼ cup (60 ml) raw coconut water, preferably fermented
½ cup (72.5 g) fresh blueberries

½ cup (33.5 g) chopped fresh kale
½ avocado
1 tablespoon (1 g) chopped fresh cilantro or parsley (optional)
1 teaspoon organic raw honey

In a food processor or high-speed blender, blend the almonds and coconut water until smooth. Add the blueberries, kale, avocado, cilantro (if using), and honey; blend until smooth. Apply 1 tablespoon (about 15 g) to your clean, dry face. Leave it on for 10 minutes, and then rinse it off with warm water.

TURN IT INTO A SMOOTHIE

I love this dual-purpose recipe. Save time and resources by making the mask as directed. Once you scoop out enough mixture for the mask, add ½ to 1 cup (120 to 235 ml) organic unsweetened coconut milk to the remaining mixture, and a handful of ice if you like your smoothie cold. Blend and enjoy!

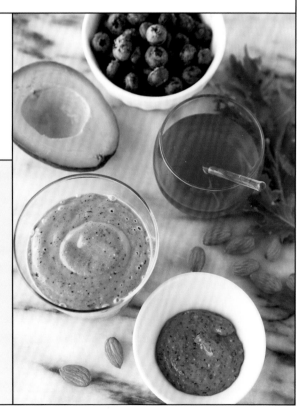

PUMPKIN MASK	With its high carotenoid antioxidant content, pumpkin is fabulous for dry or mature Sage skin (see pages 28–30). My favorite ingredients—honey, avocado, and yogurt—are included here for added benefit. This mask is hydrating and nourishing for all skin types.
	YIELD: 2 applications

2 tablespoons (31 g) organic canned pure pumpkin, or freshly cooked pumpkin 1 tablespoon (9 g) avocado	½ teaspoon organic raw honey ½ teaspoon Greek yogurt, or whole-fat yogurt

In a blender or food processor, blend the pumpkin, avocado, honey, and yogurt. Apply to your face and let sit for 15 minutes. Rinse with warm water.

BODY TREATMENTS

While the face is the main focus of this chapter, I also include a few of my favorite DIY body treatments. Don't forget to do a patch test on your forearm before applying anything to your entire body.

EXFOLIATING BODY POLISH	This natural body exfoliator is great for removing dead skin. It should not be used on the face or on broken skin (with open wounds and eruptions), as it can be irritating.
	YIELD: 6 applications

½ cup (100 g) cooked brown rice ½ cup (120 ml) organic unsweetened coconut milk	¼ cup (60 g) brown sugar

In a blender, pulverize the rice. Add the coconut milk and brown sugar; blend until smooth. Massage the mask onto your skin where there is a buildup of dead skin (such as your back, abdomen, chest, arms, legs, and feet) for about 5 minutes. Remove the mask in a warm shower.

HYDRATING BODY OIL

This natural hydrator is great for dry skin. Avoid using it on your face if you're an Olivia skin type (see pages 25–26).

YIELD: 12 applications

1 (400 IU) vitamin E capsule
½ cup (120 ml) almond oil

¼ cup (60 ml) avocado oil
5 to 10 drops ylang-ylang essential oil, or lavender essential oil

Puncture the vitamin E capsule and squeeze its contents into a small bowl. Stir in the almond, avocado, and ylang-ylang oils. Massage over your entire body. You can leave this oil on or shower it off with warm water after 10 to 20 minutes.

OATMEAL BODY SCRUB

This natural body scrub is great for removing dead skin. It should not be used on the face or on skin with open wounds and eruptions. It is more hydrating than the Exfoliating Body Polish (see left) because of the oil and oats.

YIELD: 10 to 12 applications

¾ cup (52 g) organic whole raw oats
¼ cup (60 ml) almond oil, or sesame seed oil

¼ cup (60 g) brown sugar

In a blender or food processor, blend the oats, oil, and brown sugar. Massage over your entire body (avoiding the face) with your fingers for about 5 minutes. Rinse off in a warm shower.

OATMEAL BATH	This body treatment is a great option for itchy, inflamed, and irritated skin to help soothe and nourish. It's especially soothing for Emmett-types (see pages 27–28), whose skin issues often cover various areas of the body.
	YIELD: 1 bath

1 to 2 cups (156 to 312 g) organic whole raw oats

Draw a warm, not hot, bath. Place the oats in a thin sock, bandana, or other thin piece of cotton fabric and secure with a rubber band or string. Place the oat sachet in the bath, step in, and relax. Squeeze the sock periodically to release the skin-nourishing oats into the water.

Enjoy this healing soak for at least 10 minutes. No need to rinse your body afterward unless it feels sticky or uncomfortable. You can even rub the oatmeal over your skin, if desired.

CHAMOMILE, ELDERFLOWER, AND ROSE TEA HERBAL BATH	This tea bath is relaxing and soothing for all skin types. If you have an allergy to any of these herbs, do not use this recipe.
	YIELD: 1 bath

¼ cup (8 g) loose chamomile tea   ¼ cup (8 g) loose rose tea
¼ cup (8 g) loose elderflower tea

Fill a thin sock or thin piece of cotton fabric with the loose teas and secure with a rubber band or string. Run a very warm bath, and place the herbal tea sachet in the bath under the running water. Squeeze the bag to help release the flowers' healing properties.

Step in, relax, and soak for at least 15 minutes. No need to rinse your body afterward.

CHAPTER 10

Healthy Habits for Clean Skin

If you're here, you've completed the two-week program and are happy with your skin's healthy appearance. Congratulations! Your skin should feel cleaner from within—and your external appearance will reflect that change with healthy, naturally youthful-looking skin. Your skin will have an enhanced microbiome as well, and be healthier and appear more radiant. Let's talk about what's next.

CLEAN PLATE

You're ready to move to the next stage, which includes the reintroduction phase followed by ongoing lifestyle habits to ensure your skin continues to have that healthy glow. The two-week program helps you identify which foods promote skin health, while the reintroduction phase aims to discover which foods may trigger unwanted symptoms. The end of the two-week program is a great time to recheck your symptoms to see which have disappeared and make note to see which continue. If you took my *Skin Quiz* after reading chapter 1, you may want to take it again to see how your answers compare: TheSkinQuiz.com.

Some people follow the clean plate recommendations indefinitely because they enjoy the diet and the results they see. It is healthy and safe to stay on this food plan long term, if you choose. Most people, though, start to miss foods they eliminated during the two-week program. We'll discuss how to reintroduce

SYMPTOM RECHECK

- ▸ Review the symptom checklist (see page 71). Has your score changed?

- ▸ What symptoms have you had?

- ▸ What symptoms have disappeared?

- ▸ What is different?

- ▸ How is your skin? Is it clearer? Brighter?

- ▸ Do you have more energy?

- ▸ Did you lose any weight?

- ▸ How is your mood?

- ▸ Is your focus and concentration different?

- ▸ How is your digestion?

those foods in a way that allows you to watch for changes in your skin and discover important aspects of your ongoing food plan.

REINTRODUCTION PHASE

The reintroduction phase helps you modify a food plan based on your unique needs. You can learn a great deal about your reaction to foods, including *how your skin reacts* when you eat certain things. Often, people are unaware of improvements until those symptoms start to return during this phase; or they never realized the connection between a symptom they experienced and a food they were eating until they eliminate that food. By reintroducing items in a systematic way, you can easily determine which are safe for your skin and which ones trigger internal and external health problems.

For your menu plan, follow the recommendations in chapter 3. Once you have reintroduced all foods previously eliminated and know which ones are triggers, you can avoid those and substitute healthier choices.

Here are the steps for reintroducing foods:

1. Choose one food you have eliminated during the two-week program and eat that food for two to three days. Watch for any symptoms or reactions. It's best to start with a food you do not think will cause any reactions. Do not eat any specific food you know you are allergic to. For best results, eat the selected food as part of at least two meals per day.

2. If you have a reaction, stop eating that food and wait until all symptoms are gone before reintroducing the next food.

3. Keep track of your reactions by writing them down.

4. If you have no reaction after two to three days, reintroduce the next food.

5. Continue until all foods have been reintroduced.

What's next for your clean plate? I suggest you consider the two-week program part of your ongoing health plan. I usually recommend that my patients do this program once or twice per year (or more often as needed) to help reset their lifestyle habits and clear their skin from within. You'll likely find the next time you do the two-week program is even easier than the first time! In the meantime:

▸ Most likely, you will not react to your food triggers forever, but it's best to avoid or limit them for at least three to six months.

▸ Limit or avoid caffeine, alcohol, and sugar because of their dehydrating and inflammatory effects.

▸ As much as possible, make your own food instead of eating processed food that may seem more convenient.

▸ Continue a nutrient-rich, microbiome-enhancing, and optimally balanced diet using the recipes in this book and choosing from the ten food and drink categories outlined in chapter 3 (see page 54).

NOTES ABOUT FOOD REINTRODUCTION

▸ If you have seven days or fewer to reintroduce all the eliminated foods, focus on the ones you think are the most likely to be triggers. If you don't know, focus on the most common reactive foods: *dairy*, *gluten*, and *sugar*.

▸ Continue to use the recipes from this book.

▸ If you accidently introduce more than one food and have a reaction, make note of the foods. Cut out those foods and reintroduce them again at a later date (after your reaction is gone).

▸ If you cannot determine your reactive foods, consider having food intolerance testing done. Look for a licensed naturopathic physician or functional medicine doctor who can run a full food intolerance blood panel. With one blood draw, practitioners can test for more than ninety-five different foods.

▸ Processed foods, caffeine, sugar, and alcohol are not good for the body, but some people tolerate them better than others. If you miss them, these foods can be reintroduced similarly to the others. Use caution when reintroducing them, though, as some people experience strong reactions, such as rapid heart rate. These substances are best reintroduced last. Choose the cleanest and least-processed sources possible, and enjoy them in moderation.

▸ An occasional dose of caffeine is okay for some, but consuming it throughout the day keeps our body in a state of stress, which negatively affects our neurotransmitters and adrenals.

▸ If you react negatively to alcohol, avoid it—it might be causing some of your health concerns.

CLEAN SLATE

When it comes to what you put on your body, you do *not* want to reintroduce the toxic personal care products you used before the two-week program. At this point, you've likely found natural personal care products and DIY skin care recipes you enjoy. If you're still searching, or you prefer to purchase skin care products, there are ways to identify products that are both natural and effective. I call this the science of natural beauty.

THE SCIENCE OF NATURAL BEAUTY

After years of research and clinical experience, I have discovered that natural products *can* work, *if* they're made correctly. We have the science and technology to have clean, non-toxic ingredients that are effective in helping keep skin free of breakouts, inflammation, and premature aging. Consider these factors when choosing natural and effective products.

1. Free of toxins. Covered extensively in chapter 4, you now know the top toxic ingredients to avoid because of their hormone-disrupting and other harmful effects. Refer to that list (see pages 77–79), and visit the Campaign for Safe Cosmetics website for other valuable new research and additional ingredients to avoid.

2. Contain key nutrients in their active, pure form. More research has been completed on natural ingredients than ever before. We know certain ingredients, such as green tea extract, CoQ10, and vitamin C, offer tremendous skin benefits. Choose skin care with well-balanced ingredients and potent forms of natural actives.

3. pH balanced toward mild acidity. As discussed, our skin's exterior has a naturally mild acidic environment (a pH level of about 4 to 4.5) that helps our skin stay hydrated and healthy. Cleansers and other skin care products with a higher pH (generally over 5.5) may dry your skin, making it more prone to infections, outbreaks, and premature aging. If your cleansers make suds or foam with water, they are likely too alkaline. Check the labels or ask the manufacturers if you're suspicious about a product's pH; it should be below 5.5 so your skin microbiome can flourish.

Not all natural skin care products are made using the science of natural beauty, so it is important to look closely at ingredients and ask questions. I was determined to create skin care products that embrace all three factors, and I did with my own company and The Spa Dr. skin care line. When our skin is clear and glowing, confidence follows; and that's when our real natural beauty shines through.

To maintain your clean slate:

▸ Use skin care products based on the science of natural beauty. Check out The Spa Dr.'s Daily Essentials at Store.TheSpaDr.com.

▸ Continue DIY face treatments as needed. Continue your favorite DIY cleansers and toners daily as well. Choose an exfoliant and mask to use once a week. Remember, these homemade products have a limited shelf life. Follow directions for continued safe and effective use.

▸ Find a well-trained local esthetician who uses clean and natural skin care. Avoid practices and procedures that are abrasive or strip the skin. The key to clean, glowing skin is inner and outer nourishment to enhance both the gut and skin microbiomes. Most estheticians recommend facials every four to six weeks, but they may recommend more frequent visits when your skin needs more attention.

CLEAN BODY

You've successfully reduced toxins in your home. Continuing these avoidance practices will add to your healthy habits. Review chapter 5 for the eight ways to reduce toxins in your home and six ways to reduce toxins in your food and drinks.

After completing the two-week program, you do not need to continue the home spa cleansing techniques on a daily basis. Now that you know how to practice each one and have identified which are most helpful for your needs, perform these tasks as needed for optimal health and glowing skin. I do suggest continuing your daily exercise and taking a mineral bath, doing dry skin brushing, or applying a castor oil pack or rub at least once per month. If you notice your skin starting to worsen, you can use these tools anytime.

WHY CONTINUE DAILY EXERCISE?

Studies repeatedly detail the benefits of regular exercise, and they are endless. From glowing skin, improved body composition (less fat and more muscle), and chronic disease prevention (heart disease, diabetes, depression, osteoporosis, arthritis, and certain cancers); to greater energy, better sleep, enhanced mood, memory, and cognition; to reduced stress response and better sex drive—the list goes on and on. Most research suggests benefits can result from engaging in as few as three hours per week of exercise. I recommend that amount at a minimum.

However you can, find a way to move your body every day. Exercise is most beneficial when it involves a combination of cardio and strength training. Cardio means any activity that requires you to sustain an elevated heart rate. Just be sure you're exercising within a healthy heart rate zone. Most individuals looking for mild to moderate exercise should be able to carry on a conversation while exercising. Interval or burst training (a few minutes of high-intensity cardio followed by a brief rest period) can offer weight loss and an energy boost, among other benefits, but it's important to check with your doctor before engaging in any exercise that's new for you.

If you are working too hard, exercise can do more harm than good. Overexerting yourself may place too much strain on your heart, which will elevate stress hormones. That's not only bad for your skin but may also be life threatening. Listen to your body and rest when you need—and be transparent with your primary care doctor.

Strength training involves any exercise that implements resistance, such as weight lifting. I generally recommend people get a minimum of three days per week of strength training to improve muscle tone. For the time-crunched, interval or burst training plus cardio can offer an efficient workout in a mere fifteen minutes.

SUPPLEMENTS

While a healthy diet and lifestyle are key for a clean body, for many patients, I recommend supplements for optimal health and radiant skin. Supplements can help:

- Compensate for inadequate intake of essential nutrients through diet

- Enhance body systems to function at their maximum potential

- Compensate for genetic vulnerabilities

- Provide needed vitamins for proper metabolic reactions

- Supply essential antioxidants and liver support to counteract oxidative damage

It is essential to use the highest quality supplements. I'm picky about the supplements I carry in my practice, which is why I also developed my own supplement line. It's important to work only with practitioners and supplement manufacturers who stay on top of the latest research on the safest and most effective forms of nutrients and herbs. Not all supplements are safe, however, and some can interact with prescription medications. If you take medications, work with a licensed naturopathic physician or other doctor trained in drug and nutrient interactions.

The most important supplements for ongoing clean skin are:

1. A high-quality multivitamin and mineral supplement to provide essential nutrients for healthy skin and body.

2. Essential fatty acids in combination with a balance of omega-3s and omega-6s to reap the benefits for glowing skin.

3. Antioxidants to help reverse oxidative damage from toxins in the environment.

4. Shake mixes such as my All-In-One, or another pea or hemp protein-based shake mix without any sugar, fructose, or any of the "foods to avoid." This can help start your day on a healthy foot or provide a tasty, filling snack between meals. This is a good option for people who have limited time to prepare breakfast or snacks.

In addition to these supplements, consider continuing recommended supplements for your skin type (see chapter 6). I often recommend the following supplements to my patients for daily maintenance and glowing, naturally youthful skin, available at Store.TheSpaDr.com. You may find similar products at your local health food store or naturopathic physician's clinic.

- All-In-One Daily Shake

- Daily Nutrients Packets

- Hair, Skin, and Nails Support

- Collagen Complete

- Vitamin C Fizz

- Astaxanthin + Omega Krill

- Microbiome Builder

THE SEVEN KEY HABITS FOR HEALTHY LIVING

1. Eat balanced, nutrient-rich meals, and maintain a clean plate.

2. Reduce toxins in your environment, including keeping a clean slate and clean body.

3. Strive for a balanced body, mind, and spirit for a clean mind.

4. Practice positive thinking and gratitude.

5. Exercise regularly.

6. Get adequate sleep and relaxation.

7. Develop positive relationships and interact with your community.

The stress-busting and emotion-soothing techniques you learned in chapter 5 will also help with ongoing hormone balancing and health-promoting benefits for clean skin from within. Choose your favorites from the "Six Practices for a Clean Mind" (see pages 94–96), and practice them daily. You may find that modified versions work better for you or you prefer a different technique altogether. Whatever your choice, stay dedicated to its practice so you're ready for what life throws at you.

I have studied healthy habits for years and realize this is what truly makes a difference in our health. The two-week program is excellent for pushing the reset button, but it's up to your daily practices to maintain the benefits.

When you make the choice to continue these healthy habits, you're telling your body and mind that your health is important. With wellness in hand, you can achieve more in your life. In addition to achieving and maintaining clean and glowing skin, you can reach goals you may have thought impossible. You'll have more energy and focus to take your life to the next level; you may even notice that your relationships improve. Success is at your fingertips, ready whenever you choose to focus on it.

Neuroscientists once believed the brain was unchangeable after childhood. Now we know the human brain is malleable and adapts with experience. We can establish new habits, which lead to new thinking. We need new thinking to create new neural pathways. That means we need to do things differently. When we change things, our

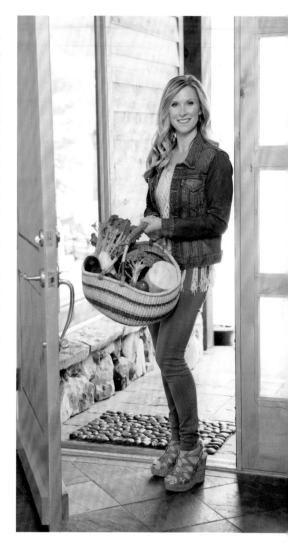

brains create new circuits that make it possible to create lasting healthy habits. Completing the two-week program helps achieve this. If, however, you are struggling to make a long-term change, consider these tips for developing a new habit:

1. Do it a different way. By doing something differently from the way you usually do it, your mind must pause long enough to make a healthier choice. Consider using a different hand or doing something upside down.

2. Change your relationship to your environment. Become aware of the environment in which you indulge in unhealthy habits. How does it support your ritual? What are the triggers? How can you change the environment to support healthier choices? If you realize your sofa is where you usually crash with a snack while watching TV, think of sitting in an armchair instead.

3. Find substitutions when needed. Another way to short-circuit habits that limit your health is to find satisfying substitutes. Choose a habit you want to change, then find a reasonable replacement. For example, if you drink sugary drinks, you may find flavoring sparkling mineral water with fresh berries, cucumber, or lime makes a satisfying substitute.

I know you will encounter hurdles, big and small. If you slip up, get up, brush it off, and get back on track. I've provided resources for support when you need it. On the right, you will find websites to help find a practitioner, online tools such as my such as my free online skin quiz (TheSkinQuiz.com), and other resources to help you stay on track.

Remember, life is a journey, and you are at the helm. I'm dedicated to helping you achieve vibrant health, glowing skin, natural beauty, and the confidence that comes with them.

I continue to provide a bounty of support for you on my website (TheSpaDr.com) through podcasts, blogs, and additional resources.

Resources

SKIN TYPE

To discover your skin type, and other valuable resources, go to TheSkinQuiz.com.

ONLINE PROGRAM

For an online version of the two-week program in this book, visit Dr. Cates's online Clear Skin Solution program at TheSpaDr.com/clearskin.

SKIN CARE

To order Dr. Cates's recommended skin care and supplements, visit Store.TheSpaDr.com

To learn more about harmful skin care ingredients, go to safecosmetics.org.

NATUROPATHIC MEDICINE

Want to learn more about naturopathic medicine? Go to naturopathic.org.

PRACTITIONERS

Looking for a practitioner in your area? For a naturopathic doctor such as Dr. Cates, go to Naturopathic.org and click "Find a Doctor" in the overhead tab.

For a functional medicine doctor, go to FunctionalMedicine.org, and enter your location to find a practitioner near you.

References

JOURNAL ARTICLES

Adebamowo, C.A., D. Spiegelman, C.S. Berkey, F.W. Danby, H.H. Rockett, G.A. Colditz, W.C. Willett, and M.D. Holmes. "Milk Consumption and Acne in Teenaged Boys." *Journal of the American Academy of Dermatology* 58, no. 5 (May 2008): 787–93. Epub January 14, 2008. doi:10.1016/j.jaad.2007.08.049.

Alkaabi, J.M., B. Al-Dabbagh, S. Ahmad, H.F. Saadi, S. Gariballa, and M.A. Ghazali. "Glycemic Indices of Five Varieties of Dates in Healthy and Diabetic Subjects." *Nutrition Journal* 10, no. 59 (May 2011). doi.org/10.1186/1475-2891-10-59.

Al-Shobaili, H.A. "Oxidants and Anti-Oxidants Status in Acne Vulgaris Patients with Varying Severity." *Annals of Clinical and Laboratory Science* 44, no. 2 (Spring 2014): 202–7. PubMed PMID: 24795060.

Amer, M., and M. Metwalli. "Topical Liquiritin Improves Melasma." *International Journal of Dermatology* 39, no. 4 (April 2000): 299–301. PubMed PMID: 10809983.

Barp, L., C. Kornauth, T. Wuerger, M. Rudas, M. Biedermann, A. Reiner, N. Concin, and K. Grob. "Mineral Oil in Human Tissues, Part I: Concentrations and Molecular Mass Distributions." *Food and Chemical Toxicology* 72 (October 2014): 312–21. Epub April 26, 2014. doi:10.1016/j.fct.2014.04.029.

Berardesca, E., N. Cameli, C. Cavallotti, J.L. Levy, G.E. Piérard, and G. de Paoli Ambrosi. "Combined Effects of Silymarin and Methylsulfonylmethane in the Management of Rosacea: Clinical and Instrumental Evaluation." *Journal of Cosmetic Dermatology* 7, no. 1 (March 2008): 8–14. doi:10.1111/j.1473-2165.2008.00355.x.

Bissett, D.L., J.E. Oblong, and C.A. Berge. "Niacinamide: A B Vitamin that Improves Aging Facial Skin Appearance." *Dermatologic Surgery* 31, no. 7, Part 2 (July 2005): 860–5; discussion 865. PubMed PMID: 16029679.

Bouilly-Gauthier, D., C. Jeannes, Y. Maubert, L. Duteil, C. Queille-Roussel, N. Piccardi, C. Montastier, et al. "Clinical Evidence of Benefits of a Dietary Supplement Containing Probiotic and Carotenoids on Ultraviolet-Induced Skin Damage." *British Journal of Dermatology* 163, no. 3 (September 2010): 536–43. Epub July 26, 2010. doi:10.1111/j.1365-2133.2010.09888.x.

Bowe, W.P., and A.C. Logan. "Acne Vulgaris, Probiotics, and the Gut-Brain-Skin Axis—Back to the Future?" *Gut Pathogens* 3, no. 1 (2011). doi.org/10.1186/1757-4749-3-1.

Burlando, B., and L. Cornara. "Honey in Dermatology and Skin Care: A Review." *Journal of Cosmetic Dermatology* 12, no. 4 (December 2013): 306–13. doi:10.1111/jocd.12058. Review.

Chang, Y.S., M.K. Trivedi, A. Jha, Y.F. Lin, L. Dimaano, and M.T. García-Romero. "Synbiotics for Prevention and Treatment of Atopic Dermatitis: A Meta-Analysis of Randomized Clinical Trials." *JAMA Pediatrics* 170, no. 3 (March 2016): 236–42. doi:10.1001/jamapediatrics.2015.3943.

Concin, N., G. Hofstetter, B. Plattner, C. Tomovski, K. Fiselier, K. Gerritzen, S. Semsroth, et al. "Evidence for Cosmetics as a Source of Mineral Oil Contamination in Women." *Journal of Women's Health* 20, no. 11 (November 2011): 1713–9. Epub October 4, 2011. doi:10.1089/jwh.2011.2829.

Craig, S.A. "Betaine in Human Nutrition." *American Journal of Clinical Nutrition* 80, no. 3 (September 2004): 539–49. Review. PubMed PMID: 15321791.

Danby, F.W. "Nutrition and Acne." *Clinics in Dermatology* 28, no. 6 (November–December 2010): 598–604. doi:10.1016/j.clindermatol.2010.03.017.

Darbre, P.D., A. Aljarrah, W.R. Miller, N.G. Coldham, M.J. Sauer, and G.S. Pope. "Concentrations of Parabens in Human Breast Tumours." *Journal of Applied Toxicology* 24, no. 1 (January–February 2004): 5–13. PubMed PMID: 14745841.

Davis, E.C., and V.D. Callender. "Postinflammatory Hyperpigmentation: A Review of the Epidemiology, Clinical Features, and Treatment Options in Skin of Color." *The Journal of Clinical and Aesthetic Dermatology* 3, no. 7 (2010): 20–31.

De Groot, A.C., and M. Veenstra. "Formaldehyde-Releasers in Cosmetics in the U.S.A. and in Europe." *Contact Dermatitis* 62 (2010): 221–24. doi:10.1111/j.1600-0536.2009.01623.x.

Diamanti-Kandarakis, E., J.P. Bourguignon, L.C. Giudice, R. Hauser, G.S. Prins, A.M. Soto, R.T. Zoeller, and A.C. Gore. "Endocrine-Disrupting Chemicals: An Endocrine Society Scientific Statement." *Endocrine Reviews* 30, no. 4 (2009): 293–342. doi:10.1210/er.2009-0002.

Duarte, T.L., M.S. Cooke, and G.D. Jones. "Gene Expression Profiling Reveals New Protective Roles for Vitamin C in Human Skin Cells." *Free Radical Biology and Medicine* 46, no. 1 (January 2009): 78–87. Epub October 9, 2008. doi:10.1016/j.freeradbiomed.2008.09.028.

Fisk, W.A., H.A. Lev-Tov, A.K. Clark, and R.K. Sivamani. "Phytochemical and Botanical Therapies for Rosacea: A Systematic Review." *Phytotherapy Research* 29, no. 10 (October 2015): 1439–51. Epub August 14, 2015. doi:10.1002/ptr.5432. Review.

Fowler Jr., J.F., H. Woolery-Lloyd, H. Waldorf, and R. Saini. "Innovations in Natural Ingredients and Their Use in Skin Care." *Journal of Drugs in Dermatology* 9, no. 6 Supplement (June 2010): s72–81; quiz s82–3. PubMed PMID: 20626172.

Fu, J., G. Hillebrand, P. Raleigh, J. Li, M. Marmor, V. Bertucci, P. Grimes, S. Mandy, M. Perez, S. Weinkle, and J. Kaczvinsky. "A Randomized, Controlled Comparative Study of the Wrinkle Reduction Benefits of a Cosmetic Niacinamide/Peptide/Retinyl Propionate Product Regimen vs. a Prescription 0·02% Tretinoin Product Regimen." *The British Journal of Dermatology* 162, no. 3 (2010): 647–54. doi.org/10.1111/j.1365-2133.2009.09436.x.

Giovannini, D., A. Gismondi, A. Basso, L. Canuti, R. Braglia, A. Canini, F. Mariani, et al. "Essential Oil Exerts Antibacterial and Anti-Inflammatory Effect in Macrophage Mediated Immune Response to Staphylococcus Aureus." *Immunological Investigations* 45, no. 1 (2016): 11–28. doi:10.3109/088201 39.2015.1085392.

Gupta, M., V.K. Mahajan, K.S. Mehta, and P.S. Chauhan. "Zinc Therapy in Dermatology: A Review." *Dermatology Research and Practice* 2014 (2014). doi.org/10.1155/2014/709152.

Hanifin, J.M., and M.L. Reed. "Eczema Prevalence and Impact Working Group. A Population-Based Survey of Eczema Prevalence in the United States." *Dermatitis* 18, no. 2 (June 2007): 82–91. PubMed PMID: 17498413.

Hay, R.J., N.E. Johns, H.C. Williams, I.W. Bolliger, R.P. Dellavalle, D.J. Margolis, R. Marks, et al. "The Global Burden of Skin Disease in 2010: An Analysis of the Prevalence and Impact of Skin Conditions." *Journal of Investigative Dermatology* 134, no. 6 (June 2014): 1527–34. Epub October 28, 2013. doi:10.1038/jid.2013.446.

Ikeno, H., T. Tochio, H. Tanaka, and S. Nakata. "Decrease in Glutathione May Be Involved in Pathogenesis of Acne Vulgaris." *Journal of Cosmetic Dermatology* 10, no. 3 (September 2011): 240–4. doi:10.1111/j.1473-2165.2011.00570.x.

Jones, J., W. Mosher, and K. Daniels "Current Contraceptive Use in the United States, 2006–2010, and Changes in Patterns of Use Since 1995." *National Health Statistics Reports*. (October 2012). www.cdc.gov/nchs/data/nhsr/nhsr060.pdf.

Jung, J.Y., H.H. Kwon, J.S. Hong, J.Y. Yoon, M.S. Park, M.Y. Jang, and D.H. Suh. "Effect of Dietary

Supplementation with Omega-3 Fatty Acid and Gamma-Linolenic Acid on Acne Vulgaris: A Randomised, Double-Blind, Controlled Trial." *Acta Dermato Venereologica* 94, no. 5 (September 2014): 521–5. doi:10.2340/00015555-1802.

Khodaeiani, E., R.F. Fouladi, M. Amirnia, M. Saeidi, and E.R. Karimi. "Topical 4% Nicotinamide vs. 1% Clindamycin in Moderate Inflammatory Acne Vulgaris." *International Journal of Dermatology* 52, no. 8 (August 2013): 999–1004. Epub June 20, 2013. doi:10.1111/ijd.12002.

Kim, G., and J.H. Bae. "Vitamin D and Atopic Dermatitis: A Systematic Review and Meta-Analysis." *Nutrition* (February 2016): pii: S0899-9007(16)00077-0. Epub ahead of print. doi:10.1016/j.nut.2016.01.023.

Kim, H.K., H.K. Chang, S.Y. Baek, J.O. Chung, C.S. Rha, S.Y. Kim, B.J. Kim, and M.N. Kim. "Treatment of Atopic Dermatitis Associated with Malassezia Sympodialis by Green Tea Extracts Bath Therapy: A Pilot Study." *Mycobiology* 40, no. 2 (June 2012): 124–8. Epub June 29, 2012. doi:10.5941/MYCO.2012.40.2.124.

Kim, J.E., S.R. Yoo, M.G. Jeong, J.Y. Ko, and Y.S. Ro. "Hair Zinc Levels and the Efficacy of Oral Zinc Supplementation in Patients with Atopic Dermatitis." *Acta Dermato Venereologica* 94, no. 5 (September 2014): 558–62. doi:10.2340/00015555-1772.

Knott, A., V. Achterberg, C. Smuda, H. Mielke, G. Sperling, K. Dunckelmann, A. Vogelsang, et al. "Topical Treatment with Coenzyme Q10-Containing Formulas Improves Skin's Q10 Level and Provides Antioxidative Effects." *Biofactors* 41, no. 6 (November–December 2015): 383–90. doi:10.1002/biof.1239. Epub December 9, 2015.

Lambers, H., S. Piessens, A. Bloem, H. Pronk, and P. Finkel. "Natural Skin Surface pH Is on Average Below 5, Which Is Beneficial for Its Resident Flora." *International Journal of Cosmetic Science* 28, no. 5 (October 2006): 359–70. doi:10.1111/j.1467-2494.2006.00344.x.

Lee, D.E., C.S. Huh, J. Ra, I.D. Choi, J.W. Jeong, S.H. Kim, J.H. Ryu, et al. "Clinical Evidence of Effects of Lactobacillus Plantarum HY7714 on Skin Aging: A Randomized, Double Blind, Placebo-Controlled Study." *Journal of Microbiology and Biotechnology* 25, no. 12 (December 2015): 2160–8. doi:10.4014/jmb.1509.09021.

Lee, H.R., S.W. Kim, M.S. Kim, S.J. Son, J.H. Lee, and H.S. Lee. "The Efficacy and Safety of Gamma-Linolenic Acid for the Treatment of Acne Vulgaris." *International Journal of Dermatology* 53, no. 3 (March 2014): e199–200. doi:10.1111/ijd.12026. Epub May 15, 2013.

Lenoir, M., F. Serre, L. Cantin, and S.H. Ahmed. "Intense Sweetness Surpasses Cocaine Reward." *PLOS ONE* 2, no. 8 (2007): e698. http://doi.org/10.1371/journal.pone.0000698.

Liu, C.H., and H.Y. Huang. "In Vitro Anti-Propionibacterium Activity by Curcumin Containing Vesicle System." *Chemical and Pharmaceutical Bulletin* 61, no. 4 (2013): 419–25. PubMed PMID: 23546001.

Mahmood, S.N., and W.P. Bowe. "Diet and Acne Update: Carbohydrates Emerge as the Main Culprit." *Journal of Drugs in Dermatology* 13, no. 4 (April 2014): 428–35. PubMed PMID: 24719062.

Melnik, B.C. "Linking Diet to Acne Metabolomics, Inflammation, and Comedogenesis: An Update." *Journal of Clinical, Cosmetic, and Investigational Dermatology* 8 (July 2015): 371–88. doi:10.2147/CCID.S69135.

Michail, S. "The Role of Probiotics in Allergic Diseases." *Allergy, Asthma, and Clinical Immunology* 5, no.1 (October 2009): 5. doi: 10.1186/1710-1492-5-5.

Misery, L., P. Wolkenstein, J.M. Amici, R. Maghia, E. Brenaut, C. Cazeau, J.J. Voisard, and C. Taïeb. "Consequences of Acne on Stress, Fatigue, Sleep Disorders, and Sexual Activity: A Population-Based Study." *Acta Dermato Venereologica* 95, no. 4 (April 2015): 485–8. doi:10.2340/00015555-1998.

Niederer, M., T. Stebler, and K. Grob. "Mineral Oil and Synthetic Hydrocarbons in Cosmetic Lip Products." *International Journal of Cosmetic Science* 38, no. 2 (April 2016): 194–200. Epub October 7, 2015. doi:10.1111/ics.12276.

Ni, Z., Y. Mu, and O. Gulati. "Treatment of Melasma with Pycnogenol." *Phytotherapy Research* 16, no. 6 (September 2002): 567–71. PubMed PMID: 12237816.

Pan, S., C .Yuan, A. Tagmount, R.A. Rudel, J.M. Ackerman, P. Yaswen, C.D. Vulpe, and D.C. Leitman. "Parabens and Human Epidermal Growth Factor Receptor Ligand Cross-Talk in Breast Cancer Cells." *Environmental Health Perspectives* 124, no. 5 (May 2016): 563–69. http://dx.doi.org/10.1289/ehp.1409200.

Proksch, E., and H.P. Nissen. "Dexpanthenol Enhances Skin Barrier Repair and Reduces Inflammation after Sodium Lauryl Sulphate-Induced Irritation." *Journal of Dermatological Treatment* 13, no. 4 (December 2002): 173–8. PubMed PMID: 19753737.

Rachakonda, T.D., C.W. Schupp, and A.W. Armstrong. "Psoriasis Prevalence among Adults in the United States." *Journal of the American Academy of Dermatology* 70, no. 3 (March 2014): 512–16. doi:10.1016/j.jaad.2013.11.013. Epub January 2, 2014.

Saravanabhavan, G., M. Guay, É. Langlois, S. Giroux, J. Murray, and D. Haines. "Biomonitoring of Phthalate Metabolites in the Canadian Population through the Canadian Health Measures Survey (2007–2009)." *International Journal of Hygiene and Environmental Health* 216, no. 6 (November 2013): 652–61. doi:10.1016/j.ijheh.2012.12.009.

Shalita, A.R., J.G. Smith, L.C. Parish, M.S. Sofman, and D.K. Chalker. "Topical Nicotinamide Compared with Clindamycin Gel in the Treatment of Inflammatory Acne Vulgaris." *International Journal of Dermatology* 34, no. 6 (June 1995): 434–7. PubMed PMID: 7657446.

Sienkiewicz, M., A. Głowacka, K. Poznańska-Kurowska, A. Kaszuba, A. Urbaniak , and E. Kowalczyk. "The Effect of Clary Sage Oil on Staphylococci Responsible for Wound Infections." *Advances in Dermatology and Allergology/Postępy Dermatologii i Alergologii* 32, no. 1 (2015): 21–26. doi.org/10.5114/pdia.2014.40957.

Volkova, L.A., I.L. Khalif, and I.N. Kabanova. "Impact of the Impaired Intestinal Microflora on the Course of Acne Vulgaris." *Klinicheskaia Meditsina* 79, no. 6 (2001): 39–41. PubMed PMID: 11525176.

Wu, J. "Anti-Inflammatory Ingredients." *Journal of Drugs in Dermatology* 7, no. 7 Supplement (July 2008): s13–6. PubMed PMID: 18681154.

Zeichner, J.A. "The Efficacy and Tolerability of a Fixed Combination Clindamycin (1.2%) and Benzoyl Peroxide (3.75%) Aqueous Gel in Adult Female Patients with Facial Acne Vulgaris." *Journal of Clinical Aesthetic Dermatology* 8, no. 4 (April 2015): 21–5. PubMed PMID: 26060514; PubMed Central PMCID: PMC4456801.

Zink, A., and C. Traidl-Hoffmann. "Green Tea in Dermatology—Myths and Facts." *Journal of the German Society of Dermatology* 13, no. 8 (August 2015): 768–75. Epub July 14, 2015. doi:10.1111/ddg.12737.

WEB PAGES AND ARTICLES

American Academy of Dermatology. "American Academy of Dermatology Issues New Guidelines of Care for Acne Treatment." February 2016. www.aad.org/media/news-releases/acne-guidelines.

Campaign for Safe Cosmetics. "Carcinogens in Cosmetics." July 2014. www.safecosmetics.org/get-the-facts/chemicals-of-concern/known-carcinogens/.

Environmental Health Perspectives. "Phthalates and Childhood Body Fat: Study Finds No Evidence of Obesogenicity." doi:10.1289/ehp.124-A78.

Euromonitor Research. "Beauty and Personal Care Trends Presented at In-Cosmetics Asia." December 2014. blog.euromonitor.com/2014/12/beauty-and-personal-care-trends-opportunities-for-the-future.html.

EWG and the Campaign for Safe Cosmetics. "Not So Sexy: Hidden Chemicals in Perfume and Cologne." May 2010. www.ewg.org/research/not-so-sexy.

EWG.org. "Teen Girls' Body Burden of Hormone-Altering Cosmetics Chemicals." September 2008. www.ewg.org/research/teen-girls-body-burden-hormone-altering-cosmetics-chemicals.

EWG's Skin Deep. "Top Tips for Safer Products." May 2016. www.ewg.org/skindeep/top-tips-for-safer-products/.

Harvard Health Publications. "Giving Thanks Can Make You Happier." November 2011. www.health.harvard.edu/healthbeat/giving-thanks-can-make-you-happier.

Mayo Clinic. "Omega-3 Fatty Acids, Fish Oil, Alpha-Linolenic Acid." November 2013. www.mayoclinic.org/drugs-supplements/omega-3-fatty-acids-fish-oil-alpha-linolenic-acid/dosing/hrb-20059372.

NTP (National Toxicology Program). *Report on Carcinogens*, 13th ed. Research Triangle Park, NC: U.S. Department of Health and Human Services, Public Health Service, 2014. http://ntp.niehs.nih.gov/pubhealth/roc/roc13/.

Vitamin D Council. "How Do I Get the Vitamin D My Body Needs?" May 2016. www.vitamindcouncil.org/about-vitamin-d/how-do-i-get-the-vitamin-d-my-body-needs/.

Acknowledgments

I want to acknowledge, first, my three children—Tiernan, Truan, and Thalia—for their enthusiasm when testing my recipes and, most importantly, for being my biggest teachers in life. Add to that my partner, Christian Gennerman, for all his loving support, and his son, Caden, for his courageous enthusiasm trying a variety of recipes.

I am also grateful to my parents—Gwen and Bill Cates—for raising me on a farm, teaching me how to enjoy whole foods, and introducing me to natural medicine.

This brings me to my gratitude for all my professors at the National University of Natural Medicine who provided me with a solid foundation for my naturopathic medicine practice.

I also want to thank Chef Jarrett Schwartz for his help with recipe tweaks, making them even more delicious.

To my skin care superstar friends, I owe great thanks to Karen Sinclair Drake for expanding my understanding of skin care ingredients and well-balanced blends, as well as her support in helping formulate The Spa Dr.'s Daily Essentials skin care system. Thanks also go to holistic esthetician Rachael Pontillo for her valuable feedback on the DIY skin care recipes.

Finally, thank you to the other experts and my patients who have helped shape my understanding and viewpoint of skin care over the past two decades.

About the Author

Dr. Trevor Cates, also known as "The Spa Dr.," is an internationally recognized naturopathic doctor and the first woman licensed as a naturopathic doctor in the state of California. Former Governor Arnold Schwarzenegger twice appointed Dr. Cates to California's Bureau of Naturopathic Medicine Advisory Council. She has worked with world-renowned spas and sees patients in her private practice in Park City, Utah, with a focus on graceful aging and glowing skin.

She has been featured on *The Doctors, Extra, First for Women,* and on the mindbodygreen website and is host of *THE SPA DR.* podcast. Dr. Cates believes the key to healthy skin is inner *and* outer nourishment with nontoxic ingredients.

Dr. Cates's The Spa Dr. skin care and supplement lines are formulated with natural and organic ingredients designed to help you achieve the clean and natural path to confidence and beautiful skin. Visit TheSpaDr.com/specialoffer for more information.

Index